BAGs Around the World

Thoughts and words offering solace & inspiration to
ignite the human spirit

by
Jo-Ann L. Tremblay

Ottawa Canada
Go Figure Creations
www.jo-annltremblay.com
Blog: joannltremblay.wordpress.com
facebook: Jo-Ann L. Tremblay
Twitter: @joanntremblay

1st Edition

First Go Figure Creations electronic edition October 23, 2016

Amazon.com edition October 23, 2016

Designed by Go Figure Creations

Cover design copyright © 2016 Go Figure Creations

Cover Photo copyright © 2016 Jo-Ann L. Tremblay

Photography by Jo-Ann L. Tremblay

Author's Photo by Mark J. R. Henderson

ISBN-13: 978-0-9809009-3-4

DEDICATION

This book is dedicated to ALL people world wide. We are on a remarkable journey. Embrace the adventure, and may you play, love and laugh, as you live life to the fullest, in spite of it all.

Table of Contents

Table of Contents

Table of Contents

Table of Contents

Fellowship of the Bag

Bags Around The World holds the promise of inspiration for those of us who on some days feel hope is all we have. Many ostomates, their family and friends find a home in knowing we are not alone. There are legions of us worldwide, we are members of the *"fellowship of the bag"*.

We have faced our share of sadness, loneliness, pain, trauma, and the awe we experience as we are graced with another chance, our bonus life. We are learning to adapt to our new body, our new normal. Together our strength creates a powerful yet gentle and uplifting wind intent on supporting, and at times when necessary, carrying one another. Our camaraderie is the inspiration that ignites our human spirit.

When I began my journey towards ostomy awareness and advocacy my desire was to generate and create a blog that would serve the ostomy (primarily), and the non-ostomy community. Each blog post is a choice of the possibilities that comes from questions of what is, what could be, and what will be a contribution to our ostomy world.

Throughout my life I have never entertained the thought that I would ever create change in the world. I have instead set out to create a difference in my life and in someone else's life. My experiences are the lanterns that shine the light along the path of life and illuminate my understanding that *ALL*, no matter who we are, can make a difference. It is my hope that **THE**

OSTOMY FACTOR blog, through a thought, a word, a sentence or a full post, has touched you the reader in some way, and has sparked a meaningful difference in your life.

Thank you for your continued blog readership, personal comments contributions, and support of **THE OSTOMY FACTOR**. Enjoy and remember, *everyone you meet has a story to tell.*

Introduction

Welcome to *Bags Around The World*. I am an ostomate and Percy is my stoma. We are one of legions of ostomates worldwide, we are members of the *"fellowship of the bag"*.

When Percy my stoma was created there was instantly a rupture in the normal course of my life. It was an emergency life-saving surgery, and I was left stunned into incomprehension. Ostomy had never been discussed, I didn't really know what an ostomy was, I only knew some folks eliminate in a pouch, whatever that meant. The tragedy of the illness that brought me to that point, and the physical alternation that would be permanent, sent me on a turbulent intellectual, emotional and physical, pilgrimage to discover the meanings in and of my life.

Initially I felt the painful experience had damaged me. I was broken physically, emotionally, intellectually, and my human spirit seemed shattered. I was lost at the very moment I began the journey to my new normal, my bonus life.

Although my colon was no longer connected, my whole being began to reconnect as I began to recount and then discover what is important to me, what is meaningful, and what is not meaningful anymore. The pain revealed things not otherwise had ever been seen by me. When I arrived at the core of my pain it marked the moment when what was unseen in normal circumstances became more visible.

With each new pain, tragedy, joy and life triumph experienced during the bonus times of this life journey, I am alive. With each experience I am given the opportunity to expand and enhance the depth of meaning of the beauty of life. The beauty of living life large, living every tiny piece of intimacy, and living life to the fullest in spite of it all.

Committed to ostomy awareness and advocacy, my stoma Percy and I are moving forward with creating and posting **THE OSTOMY FACTOR** blogs. Blogs are usually a discussion or informational site published on the World Wide Web, available for people around the world to read and enjoy. **THE OSTOMY FACTOR** is intended to be a valuable communication tool for sharing with ostomates, caregivers, medical professionals, and non-ostomates alike.

I chose to title the blog, **THE OSTOMY FACTOR**, as the meaning of factor is; a circumstance, fact or influence that contributes to a result or outcome. Factor, fits well with how I feel about my ostomy, and how I am required to live now.

I thought long and hard on how I could incorporate Percy into the commitment and to be active with me. And so, I have given Percy a public voice, I feel there is great value in Percy speaking stoma to stoma, as well as, stoma to ostomate. Percy is an experienced stoma on the move, writing some of the blog posts, with the clever little stoma's own humorous style.

Embracing the life of an ostomate after a lengthy illness and life saving surgery in 2011, I began my ostomy writing with the intent to share life's ups and downs mixed in with inspirational and uplifting messages.

I believe, "*Everyone you meet has a story to tell*". **THE OS-TOMY FACTOR** blogs are my stories and I invite *ALL* to share with me. Together, every story carries messages of hope as we explore the realities of life, and celebrate the triumph of the human spirit. The style of writing is accessible and con-versational, and it is my hope that the blog posts will leave you entertained, informed and feeling empowered.

BAGs Around the World, begins with my very first blog post, dated November 2012, (Chances Are), and continues ending with the December 2015 post.

May you find **THE OSTOMY FACTOR** blog posts valuable in your daily life for a chuckle, a tear, and for contemplation as you go forward in life.

ENJOY!

Year 1

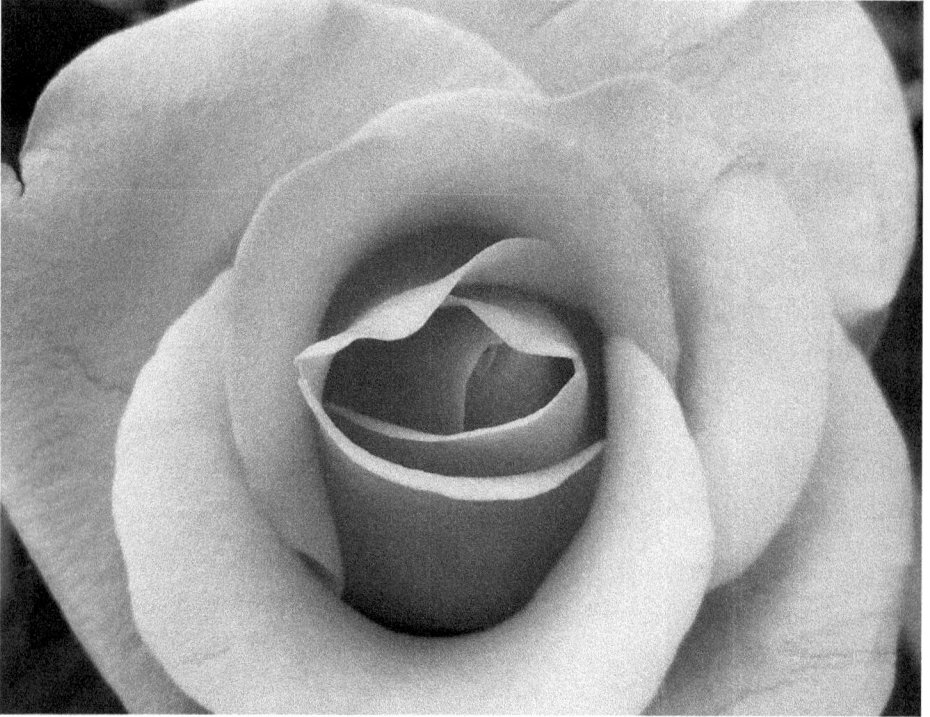

We get one life to live, yet, every day we wake up with another chance to give and receive the best we can to and from life.

It was in September of 2012, Percy and I had been working very hard as a team to recover and adjust to our new normal. Deep in my bones I felt something profound was happening. The underlying message of this feeling was; the anticipation that something great and something terrible was happening to me. There is a time in all of our lives when something important to us is lost. Then, there is the time when we really and truly notice the loss. We enter into upset, denial, we can even feel anger, and we grieve our loss. We experience the difficult moments when we remember what we lost, and we want to go back to the time before our loss for a visit. We strive to make peace with what has happened. Then, we explore what we can do about it all, so that we can come out to the other side. And so, it was time to lift my head high, and buck up.

Is my glass half full, or is it half empty? Well, my glass as it turns out is refillable.

My commitment to ostomy exploration, awareness and advocacy, was now set firmly into my heart, mind and soul. With the exception of a few, most of us need to practice, practice, and more practice to hone our skills and this is me. I learn by doing, and so with some anxiety and a great deal of enthusiasm I started the odyssey that has become **THE OSTOMY FACTOR**. An odyssey is a long intellectual and spiritual wandering and quest, that comes from the description of the travels of Homer's Odyssey. As part of my recovery and life journey going forward I created the blog series. The series that supports my commitments and my desire to connect as a member of the *fellowship of the bag*, worldwide. Part 1 of this book starts with my very first 4 blog postings, the postings that would amount to my first kick at the can, so to speak.

I endeavour to post a blog entry once a month. I am in gratitude for the folks who take the time from their busy lives to read the blog posts, and the many who sign up to receive the blog posts delivered to their computer when they are posted.

Chances Are - *November 14, 2012*

My name is Jo-Ann L. Tremblay, I am an ostomate, and my stoma's name is "Percy". Percy's name origin/meaning – British derived from latin origin, a version of a name used among the ancient Gauls. "Persius", meaning; "to penetrate the hedge".

My colostomy was created during life saving surgery July 21, 2011. It has been just over a year and my recovery is well on its way. It's time for celebrating life. It is my second chance, the bonus, the icing on the cake, the cherry on top. My first chance was amazing, my second chance incredible. Life is fragile, limited and precious. Always have had the time of my life, why not, it's the only life I thought I had. Now, with a second chance I'm having the time of my life, why not, it's the only life I know I have.

We get only one life to live, yet, every day we wake up with another chance to give and receive the best we can to and from life. They say, *"In the end, we only regret the chances we didn't take"*. Those of us who have an ostomy know what another chance is. We know we've been given another opportunity to laugh and play. We know we have another chance to suffer and cry. We know we have another crack at living and then dying. Through our rebirth we have been given the experiential mileage required to make the informed decisions necessary to make the best of life that we possibly can. **"Chances are"**, is our credo. How phenomenal is this! How gifted we are!

As we look back on the journey that brought us to the creation of our ostomies, how awful and incredible it was. At times we want to forget all of it, it has left bad stuff in our mind. The journey was jaw-dropping, amazing and horrible.

Many of us sport our ostomies in respectful silence. Let's face it, most people really don't like us talking about it–too much information they say as they cut us off in mid-sentence. Some of us are worried and embarrassed about the potential of smelling. Others are concerned about their parastomal hernia bumps, protruding out there for all the world to see. Let's face it, if we could have it any other way, we'd really rather not have a ostomy. But, the fact remains this is part of who and what we are. We are ostomates and proud of it.

Percy and I have created this blog, "**THE OSTOMY FACTOR**", for the purpose of sharing with our fellow ostomates. We have had many adventures and misadventures, as so many ostomates can relate to. Our aim is to connect with ostomates, their caregivers, the medical community, and from time to time talk stoma to stoma. Sharing with stomas is Percy's contribution. He has a sense of humour and is quite the little pooper. He's also very clever holding an EoI. in Poopology. (EoI. – **E**xperience **O**f **L**ife).

Our mission is to share the ostomates life, times, ups, down, and all arounds with the ostomy community through humour and inspiration. I have written my second book, "***Better WITH a Bag Than IN A Bag*** – *From the brink of death to recovery through humour and inspiration.* I'll keep you posted on the publication date.

Jo-Ann L. Tremblay
Ostomate
"Everyone you meet has a story to tell."

Percy & Me Are So Excited – *December 3, 2012*

It is with pleasure, we are announcing ***Better WITH a Bag Than IN a Bag – From the brink of death to recovery through humour and inspiration*** is now published and available for purchase on Amazon worldwide. We know you will enjoy reading your very own copy, and we look forward to your review feedback and comments.

Jo-Ann L. Tremblay & Percy
"Everyone you meet has a story to tell."

Shock & Awe – *December 10, 2012*

Greetings everyone, I'm Jo-Ann's stoma. When things are not going well, which happens from time to time Jo-Ann affectionately refers to me as her, "Little Pooper". I was created July 21, 2011, and I'm considered by Jo-Ann as one of her heroes. According to the Doctors she was 1 hour from certain death, and I needed to be there for her. When we awakened from the lifesaving surgery and found out I was now her outdoor plumbing, we were both shocked!

Looking back from that fateful day, the life I had known before was over. I had spent my days nestled in her warm abdomen since she was born. I was very different in those days, being attached along her large intestine, doing what I was born to do. My function was to absorb nutrients, minerals and water from the food matter, and then pass the useless waste material from Jo-Ann's body. As part of her colon, Jo-Ann and I had a lot of adventures together for many years. We travelled the World enjoying the cultural diversity of many countries through their food and cuisine. Now I must say we seemed to always find ourselves experiencing difficulty while digesting our amazing food, but life goes on and we did our best to adjust. Then in 2008, things got worse for us. You can read all about it in our book, "Better WITH a Bag Than IN a Bag"–from the brink of death to recovery through humour and inspiration.

We were researching the other day, and we found out that the word "stoma" comes from the Greek word meaning "mouth". It's actually a plural word and to be specific it means mouths. The things we find out as I adjust to my new role is amazing. It has opened a whole new world for us. In fact, recently we had the pleasure of speaking with representatives at the Colorectal Cancer Association of Canada, www.colorectal-cancer.ca. We've learned colon cancer is 90% curable if detected early. This is incredible, think of how much suffering can be avoided, how many lives can be saved. In 2011 an estimated 22,200 new cases of colon cancer were diagnosed in Canada. Close to 8,900 Canadians lost their lives that same year. Estimated new cases in the United States in 2011 were 103,170 colon cancer and 40,290 rectal cancer. Deaths in that year were 51,690 colon and rectal cancer combined.

Having a colonoscopy is one of your early detection tools. It's time to put the poop on poops out there, and on everyone's mind. Our pooper equipment needs regular check ups, no matter how uncomfortable we may feel about this.

Although Jo-Ann and I are still a little shocked as to what happened to us, we are more inclined to be in awe. Awe because we have a 2nd chance to be and do anything and everything we want. We have many more opportunities to enjoy life. Most times it seems I'm the object of Jo-Ann's humour and together we share the poop on poops. As we write our blog, I'll enjoy sharing my stoma experiences and tales. Stoma to stoma we'll explore the ups, downs, and all arounds of the world of stomas, ostomies, and the humans we stomas serve.

Percy, Eol. Poopology
Stoma
"Better With A Bag Than In A Bag"

From Percy & Me – *December 21, 2012*

With all the excitement during these days, may Christmas bring, joy and love to you that will last all year. Our special thoughts go out to you for a Happy New Year.

Year 2

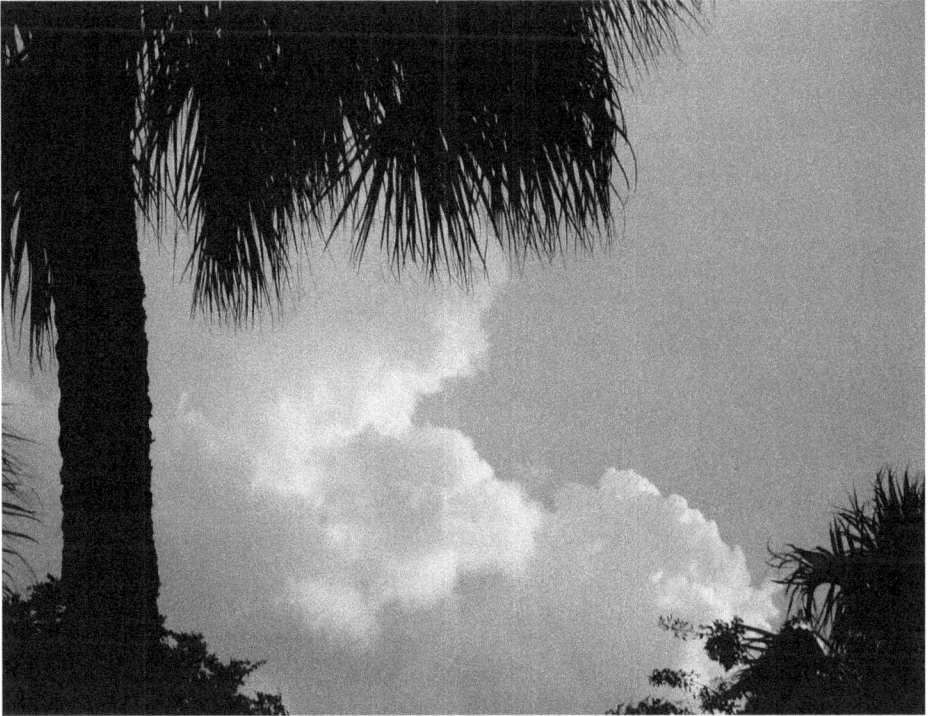

Hippocrates, the father of Western medicine, taught there is an interconnection between mind and body in healing when he emphasized that good health depends on a balance of mind, body, and environment.

Everything and everyone are connected.

As Percy and I welcomed 2013, little did we know how interesting this year would be. We continued our healing journey and every day there seemed to be a myriad of challenges and triumphs. Step by step with each challenge we reached into our bag of coping tricks, and worked hard to come up with resourceful solutions.

It is our second chance, our bonus life, and we're intent on creating and experiencing as successful of a quest for living life to the fullest as possible. And, life sure has a way of presenting some of the most delightful surprises and at times the most awful and disheartening shocks during the course of a month, a year, a lifetime. Adjusting to an altered body function takes time, patience, experiential mileage, learning, and all the while we ostomates are getting on with getting on with life in spite of it all.

It was a year of a lot of hurry up and wait. A major part of the year endured with anticipation and in preparation for the next major surgery that I was destined to undergo. It was a daunting part of my life journey, one that brought Murphy's Law to mind many times, *(If anything can go wrong, generally it does go wrong)*. Nagging at the back of my mind I felt that even if anything just cannot go wrong, it will anyway, and if everything is going right...something is wrong.

As the year progressed, I did undergo the surgery, and once and again I found myself starting a new healing journey that would take me down the path of light and dark. Living is not for wimps!

As 2013 progressed wonderful folks from around the world started connecting with Percy and I through THE OSTOMY FACTOR. They shared their special stories, experiences and thoughts with all of us and I am eternally grateful to them. We are not alone, we are a part of the community of humanity, we are ostomates. All of us are embracing life, we are reaching out to touch one another in the most supportive and profound ways. Like a strand of pearls, we don our ostomy bags as we encircle the world.

Being alive to witness the birth of children and marriages is a blessing. Being alive to travel, eat, drink and be merry is the joy of life. Then of course the universe has a sense a humour, we never know when a funny or ironic moment will present itself as with the case of goofy birds and raging toilets. Now that's an adventure of a lifetime!

Percy Gets A Dress – *January 28, 2013*

Here we are in sunny Florida, basking in the warmer than usual southwest Florida weather. Meanwhile, our family and friends at home are navigating snow covered roads, bracing themselves against a-31 Celsius windshield factor. Do wish everyone could be here with us.

Southwest Florida is known for sunshine, Everglades, white sand beaches, and some of the best bargain hunting outlets. With the wedding of one of our daughters of our blended family scheduled for the end of June, what better place to shop for a dress, I do not know.

Now it must be understood Jo-Ann is not a happy camper when shopping, even at the best of times. It's just not her thing. That's when she asks her sister-in-law Nola, to join her. Nola has a great fashion sense, loves shopping, is very patient, and gently honest about what suits or does not. So, it's off with Nola to shop.

Jo-Ann and Nola's mission if they chose to take it–was to find a "step-mother of the bride", dress that would suit Jo-Ann and camouflage me, while getting as much bang for her buck as possible.

It was early morning, (the early bird gets the worm), and already it was hot and steamy. GPS on the car dash, Nola and Jo-Ann left for the outlet.

We parked the car and took a reconnoiter of the vast parking lot, already beginning to fill, and got a sense of the lay of the land. Across the horizon as far as we could see, there were stores, stores, and more stores.

Nola excited to get started and Jo-Ann almost overwhelmed, our first stop was the outlet map. X marked the spot where we were standing, and it was time to get moving. Like a river running through a canyon we walked the ribbon of concrete between store fronts. Buildings to our right, and to our left. We were 3 on a quest for the perfect dress.

I am situated on top of a honey dew melon sized parastomal hernia, on the left side of Jo-Ann's abdomen. Jo-Ann looks about 5 months pregnant on the left side, and her right side is relatively flat. There are times when she is aware of her lop sided physique.

Under Nola's expert training, somewhat timid Jo-Ann gained confidence, and started to feel MacGyver-ish. There are resourceful fashion solutions, it's simply a matter of fashion awareness, Jo-Ann realized that she now must consider and in some cases, change her fashion style. Clothing that she liked before, for the most part do not suit her new body shape.

How to do this? Well, time to consider what draws the eye to other more flattering body parts. Next, find clothing that is constructed in such a way as to draw the eye to a decorative focal point such as; a strategically placed buckle, pleats, and so on. Looking at various fabric prints Jo-Ann realized there are patterns with various colour palettes that create a general look that once again, pulls the eye with pleasing results. And finally, Jo-Ann has learned to stay away from fabrics that cling.

It was time to enter the cool and brightly lit stores. Splitting up to cover as much ground as possible, Jo-Ann and I went to one set of racks, and Nola to another. As I mentioned, I am situated on the left side, and so my camouflage requires strategic placement. As our quest continued under the hot mid-morning sun, Nola would find a nice dress that might suit. Jo-Ann would try it on, only to realize that the focal point of that particular dress would be on the right side. Personally, my lumpy profile with a gather or a flower on the opposite side seem quite interesting to me, but, Jo-Ann and Nola certainly didn't think so. I can't tell you how many times they did this. Nola would hold up a dress and say, "Hey, this one looks great, oh, it's right handed", and they would chuckle.

Store staff even got into it, being very helpful and understanding Jo-Ann would say, "See my right side profile, this is what I look like. Now, see my left side profile, this is what I really look like". A small army of determined women in each of the stores joined us on our quest. And then the moment we all anticipated arrived. Nola found a deep purple velvet dress. It has pleats that fold diagonally from the right across the bodice and down the dress to the waist. It all meets on the left, coming together with a chiffon type material that gathers into what reminds me of a flower. From the flower, like a vertical wave, wide ribbons of chiffon drapes down to almost the hem line. This dress is elegant, with a bit of flare, it accentuates Jo-Ann's assets and camouflages me.

3 cheers, high fives and a hip hip hurray. Our mission was a success. Our quest had been filled with all of the twists, turns, challenges, and camaraderie a shopping trip offers. Our last stop would be the cash register. At home, we guesstimated the dress would probably cost us around $150.00 Canadian. But, we were at a South Florida outlet, sales abound, and who knew what the last press of the registers screen would reveal. Jo-Ann held her breath, and Nola winked as they

waited for the final sale. With a smile on her face, the store representative announced, "That will be $18.50".

Jo-Ann and Nola looked at the registers' digital screen, yes the electronic print read, $18.50. Astounding, incredible and amazing, were the thoughts that passed through Jo-Ann's mind. These thoughts translated into giggles, laughs, and a few OMG's.

As with any successful quest in life, there is always something to be learned and this one is not an exemption. I learned with a little sense, (in this case fashion sense), some resourceful-ness, and commitment, all people are beautiful just the way we are including me, just as I am.

Percy Stoma
Eol. Poopology
"Better With A Bag Than In A Bag"

Announcement – *February 13, 2013*

"Better With A Bag Than In A Bag" Jo-Ann L. Tremblay's newest book now available with Amazon.ca and Amazon.com in Kindle and paperback, will be mentioned in the "Ostomy News and Products" section of ***The Phoenix* magazine**, phoenixuoaa.org, in the March issue which mails 2/27/13.

The Phoenix magazine provides solutions to the many challenges of living with a colostomy, ileostomy, urostomy or continent diversion (j-pouch, kock pouch, etc.). From skin care to nutrition to intimacy, in-depth articles written by medical professionals, authors and ostomates show readers how to return to a full and rewarding life with an ostomy.

Percy & I Want To Share a Recent Book Review Placed On Amazon.ca – February 13, 2013:

5.0 out of 5 stars **Courageous Tale**, Feb 12 2013

By Catherine Astolfo

Format:Paperback

Jo Ann Tremblay is a brave, inspirational woman. Not only has she been through the depths of ill health and faced everything with faith and determination, but she also has the courage to take us with her on the journey. This book allows us into her thoughts as she undergoes a colostomy. It's not an easy read because it's not supposed to be. Its intimate, factual and honest.

As we age, as our parents age, we are all going to face various health challenges. Ms Tremblay's was very severe and almost killed her. In the end, her entire life changed. She has to manage a stoma appliance, whom she fondly calls Percy.

Like many people who have had to adjust to an apparatus that allows them life – although one that is transformed and suddenly dependent – Jo Ann is a hero. She adapts with humour, resolve, and love. Her family is uppermost in her mind as she struggles to get better. They love her – and as her husband Mark says, "Better with a bag than in one". She loves them enough not to give up.

I found this book sad, frightening, inspiring and joyful. I highly recommend it to anyone who is facing any kind of health challenge – or to their caregivers and loved ones. And by that I mean, all of us.

Better WITH a Bag Than IN a Bag – Book Trailer – *February 20, 2013*

Book trailer go to: youtu.be/gwrW4Xmfne4 designed and produced by Meredith Henderson, sisbroandcompany.com, take a look & if you like it share it. Enjoy

Percy Blasts Off – *February 22, 2013*

Percy and I are awaiting word as to when our next round of surgery will be. What we do know is it's scheduled for the spring of 2013. We've been in Florida for the past 6 weeks eating fresh fruit, vegetables, and taking long walks on the beach. For the most part Percy has behaved, and we had a healthy and wonderful vacation. My body and soul are nourished and refreshed, and we are ready to begin the next chapter of our life story.

In celebration, we decided a day at Kennedy Space Centre located on the Space Coast of Florida, (Atlantic Ocean side), would be our destination.

As the promotional material states; "For the last 50 years, Kennedy Space Centre has been the gateway to space exploration". It is the launch site of space science and discovery."

Our day began with multiple cinematic journeys to the end of the Earth and beyond. First, we embarked on a visual and sensory three dimensional adventure of our world that transported us beyond Earth. Together we explored the solar system.

With the end of a cosmic adventure through our galactic neighbourhood, it was off to the IMAX theatre. We gazed at the Hubble Space Telescope in 3-D, on a five story movie screen. Oh my, Mark, Percy and I, were transported through the beautiful and mysterious Universe.

From the amazing "out there", we returned closer to home as we viewed the Space Station 3-D film. From planet Earth to the International Space Station, we enjoyed the movie filmed by 25 astronauts and cosmonauts, we were amazed.

All of these experiences filled our imaginations with endless possibilities, fuelling our desire to experience space for ourselves. We wanted to see what astronauts see, and feel what they feel. It was time to know what it's like to be launched into orbit at 17,500 mph!

Feeling quite courageous we embarked on our Shuttle Launch. We were directed to a wall of equipment lockers by Kennedy Space Centre staff. Here I stowed my backpack which includes Percy's back up ostomy equipment, (I always carry this in case of a poop emergency). This should have been my 1st clue.

From here we were directed into a building with a huge multi-screen wall. We were put through an 8 ½ minute, "preflight" briefing presented by Astronaut Charlie Bolden, which is designed for the purpose of preparing us for lift off. That should have been my 2nd clue.

It was time for the experience of a lifetime. We and our fellow shuttle launch team left the pre-flight room, and lined up in our respective lines awaiting the shuttle doors to open. Capable and helpful Shuttle guides reminded the team that people with medical conditions, expectant Mothers, and so on, were welcome to experience the shuttle launch from a special room that presented all the sights and sounds of the launch, but without the physical part of the launch. Clue #3.

For the rest of us, we were congratulated and reminded we were about to experience the sights, sounds, feelings and excitement, of a vertical launch in humankind's most complex vehicle. We were about to live the thrilling launch experience of astronaut crew aboard NASA's Space Shuttle. Clue #4.

Now it was our turn to see what they have seen, feel what they've felt, and live what they've lived. The doors opened and we embarked into the simulation Shuttle cockpit. Rows of folks walked into the ship and sat in their seat. As you would find on a roller coaster ride, large metal security bars framed each seat, and we were instructed to secure our seat belts. I reached down and buckled my seat belt, and this is when I realized the belt was located right over my parastomal hernia and Percy! This is something I had not thought of and now I had a problem. How would Percy endure the Shuttle launch?

I pulled the belt lower down over my abdomen and below Percy. The belt snapped right back up over Percy. I pulled the belt up above Percy and it snapped back over Percy. Percy was caught in a situation that I had not anticipated, and I started to worry. I had put my little buddy in a potentially harmful situation. The launch was about to begin and my thoughts were with Percy. It was countdown time. I quickly slipped both my hands down and cupped Percy, hoping to protect him.

10 – 9 – 8 – 7 – 6 – 5 – 4 – 3 – 2 – 1 BLAST OFF

The noise level escalated, the visuals raced before my eyes, and the definite yet certainly **not** violent shake, rattle, and slight roll began. With both hands cupping Percy, we began to immerse ourselves into the most extraordinary and wonderful experience. With the exception of feeling G-Forces, the launch was everything we hoped it would be.

When the launch simulation ended, I released my hands and quickly unbuckled the seat belt. Percy seemed non the worse for wear. Excited, I headed for the toilette facilities for a more in-depth Percy inspection. He is absolutely fine.

I do feel my wild days of riding the roller coaster are now over. But, I fully expect to enjoy the type of rides one would find at Disney type park, for example. The Shuttle launch was our first experience of its kind since Percy's creation. Gee…ostomies affect all aspects of an ostomates life. I did not think of the seat belt and Percy's placement, and it is a good lesson to learn.

Percy and I wear our seat belt in the car at all times. On the seat belt I wear a specifically designed stoma protector. It has a velcro closure, making it easy to put on and to remove. I'm not sure if I can use this piece of equipment on all types of seat belts. We will be in investigative mode over the next while. If my current seat belt stoma protector doesn't work for all seat belts, then we'll explore how Percy can be protected by other means.

Most Important Lesson: As long as I am vigilant of Percy's needs, have the foresight to analyze situations, know/accept our limitations, and be resourceful – we will continue on our quest to live life to the fullest. We choose to live the inspired ostomates life. Ostomates have already beaten the odds, and are living proof of courage. Now that's an adventure of a lifetime.

Jo-Ann L. Tremblay
Ostomate
"Everyone you meet has a story to tell."

Hurray Up And Wait – *February 28, 2013*

Our vacation suitcases are unpacked. Refrigerator and freezer re-stocked. 2 days of relaxation and the phone rings.

"I'm hand delivering your forms to admitting Jo-Ann", said Nancy our surgeon's assistant. The next round of surgery Percy and I are expecting has begun.

2 more days, and the phone rings again. "You are booked for a pre-op appointment. Report to the Admitting desk at 7:30 a.m.", said the hospital representative.

Percy, my husband Mark and I, spent 3 hours at the hospital speaking with the admitting nurse and the anesthetist. I provided some of my blood for analysis. All the while, we anxiously awaited to hear our surgery date.

"I don't have a date written here on the form, give me a minute, and I'll make a call", said the nurse. A few minutes later she returned, "no we don't have a date yet. I can't tell you when it will be, but do know it will be soon. Meanwhile, avoid anyone with a cold, cough, sniffles, or the flu. You'll be getting a call."

So, here we are now sitting by the phone awaiting the call. My packed hospital bag stands at the ready. When the phone call comes, things will move quickly, Percy and I need to be ready.

Meanwhile, every time the phone rings, we jump. I have informed friends and family I cannot be exposed to any of their coughs, sniffles, and sneezes.

The phone volume is at it's loudest, just in case it rings and I'm in the shower. I have decided to cancel restaurant dates with friends. I've done this in the event that the folks who pre-pare the food, deliver it, or are sitting in the same room as me have a cough, sniffle or a sneeze.

The phone rings from time to time from everyone and anyone other than the hospital, (which of course I haven't heard from yet). "Patience Jo-Ann, patience." I am now inviting any of my cough-less, sniffle-less, and sneeze-less friends and family into the, as germ free as possible, confines of my home. Okay, that's it, I'm no longer concerned I will catch a cough, sniffle nor a sneeze from anyone, I'm more concerned that I'm going to catch a full blown case of cabin fever!

Hurry up and wait! Sitting here with time on my hands, no use starting anything too involved at this time because of course, I'm waiting for the phone call. I have time to think, to muse.

The youngest daughter of our blended family is an actress. I am always fascinated when I'm with her on set. Since the only job I have at those times is to observe, then observe is what I do. I am amazed to watch the drama and non-drama of hurry up and wait play out before my eyes.

Off to the side and in the dark corners ready for action, pro-duction crew patiently watch the Director and Actors do their part. When its time to change the scene the crew scramble in a flurry of coordinated activity to prepare and get everything ready to shoot the next part of the production.

This is the stage on which I have watched the hurry up and wait dance performed. It is not simple, it is coordinated, spe-cific and patient theatre. It is one of life's living truths, and there's a good lesson hidden in the scene, I'm trying to learn it.

It's my turn to dance the dance, as I wait by the phone avoiding the coughs, sniffles and sneezes as best I can. And, when it does ring, I will arabesque to the phone. I will *assemblé* as they give me the date and time of the surgery. Until then I will attitude *croisé devant* as I ballon and *ballotté* my best patience. Well, that's the plan at any rate.

Jo-Ann L. Tremblay
Ostomate
"Everyone you meet has a story to tell."

Percy Gets A Facelift – *March 11, 2013*

"Phyllis Diller's had so many facelifts, there's nothing left in her shoes" – Bob Hope

Our date with destiny has been announced. Percy and I are scheduled to undergo parastomal hernia surgery Tuesday, March 19, 2013.

A little about parastomal hernias. As soon as a stoma is constructed, a potential site of weakness in the abdominal wall is instantly produced. Parastomal hernia occurs when weakness in the abdominal wall is sufficient to permit abdominal contents, usually the intestine, to protrude through the fascial defect around the stoma and into the internal tissue, creating a bulge on the abdomen. Parastomal herniation occurs in approximately 30% of all stomas, my research indicates it is more common in colostomies than in ileostomies and urostomies

At the pre-op appointment a nurse and a doctor met with us. I signed the consent forms after reading all the things that can go wrong. Oh, that was interesting to say the least. I was given booklets such as; "Guide – Planning for my inpatient surgery", "Guide – Pain Management after surgery", "Welcome – To The Hospital Admission Information". Percy and I are informed, educated, and prepared

Our honey dew melon sized lump will undergo an interesting procedure, the small intestine repacked back in place, abdominal wall muscles will be repaired, a bio-mesh placed in order to support the abdominal wall, and in the inner abdomen Percy will be placed in a mesh hammock to provide him with the stability and support he requires. Percy's going to be quite the "lay about". The surgeon estimates the surgery will be 2 ½ to 4 hours in duration. The repair will help alleviate the discomfort and risks a parastomal hernia presents, and, if successful Henrietta Hernia will be no more.

In essence Percy is getting a facelift. Facelifts are purported to improve looks and self-confidence. With Percy permanently settled into his hammock, looking dapper and full of himself, life after surgery will be an interesting adventure indeed.

Percy and I will be in hospital, and then we expect the recovery at home to take awhile. As soon as I can sit up and concentrate long enough, we will do our best to post our blogs as often as possible throughout our recovery. Percy is anticipating writing his blogs while I'm on pain medication, hmm.......

Jo-Ann L. Tremblay & Percy
Ostomate
Percy Stoma Eol. Poopology
"Everyone you meet has a story to tell."

The Countdown Continues – *March 15, 2013*

4 days to go to major surgery. We're ready to begin the next stage of our healing journey. Spending as much time as possible partying with friends and family. Life is a grand gift for the 2nd chance at life people. The journey and the community of humanity who share it with us makes the adventure an amazing experience.

Percy would like to say, he's happy to go with the flow.

Jo-Ann L. Tremblay & Percy
Ostomate
Percy Stoma - Eol. Poopology
"Everyone you meet has a story to tell."

As Life Will Have It – *March 18, 2013*

The big day is tomorrow, and of course as my life will have it, 10 to 20 cm of snow is predicted. Stormy weather pressing in on the Ottawa Valley as the pressure of surgery presses in on us.

A blanket of snow will cover the ground as Percy and I curl up in our warm hospital blanket to weather the storms. Take care all, Percy and I would like to once again take this opportunity thank all of you for your continued support.

Jo-Ann L. Tremblay & Percy
Ostomate
Percy Stoma - Eol. Poopology
"Everyone you meet has a story to tell"

Update on Jo-Ann's Surgery By Mark Henderson (Hubby) *March 19, 2013*

After 3 hours of surgery, I am happy to report that Jo-Ann came through in great shape. The surgeon reports that all went better than expected. The parastomal hernia has been repaired, and Percy is snuggled comfortably in his new sling. She is in great spirits and recovering very comfortably (that is, the pain is being managed very well). As I left her at 8:30 PM, she was her old feisty self, joking with the nurses, and making a slew of new friends on the hospital floor. She, I, and Percy couldn't be more pleased (so far). Now the healing and re-covery begins. More tomorrow.

Wednesday, *March 20, 2013*

Everything regarding Jo-Ann's recovery is going very well. She was able to go for short walks twice today. She is an ex-traordinary trooper and has the nurses charmed (big surprise). She is still eating clear liquids only, but hopefully that will change tomorrow. Percy is passing gas very frequent-ly and making lots of noise (this is good since it means that he is progressing as well as Jo-Ann is). If the gas continues, we progress to solid food (which will let Percy do his stuff…do the thing he was born to do). Once all is working (Jo-Ann and Percy), they get to come home. More updates to follow. I have kept Jo-Ann posted regarding feedback. She sends her love and appreciates greatly hearing from you. It is much easier if we keep visitations in hospital to a minimum. I hope you un-derstand. It is so that Jo-Ann can spend her energies getting ready to come home..where you are welcome to visit anytime.

Thursday, *March 21, 2013*

It was a good day today. Jo-Ann was able to get up and walk several times. The surgeon was able to allow her solid food as of 6 PM this evening thanks to Percy gettin' the job done. Pain management is going well, although because of the mesh inserted to repair the hernia, the surgeon indicated that there would be a higher level of pain during the healing process. Jo-Ann, as always, is insisting that the pain is nothing she can't handle, although I see her wince once in a while (which is unusual for her). All in all things are proceeding according to Hoyle. I am keeping her apprised regarding the many messages you have been sending. These are much appreciated. She sends you all her love. Stay tuned...

Friday, *March 22, 2013*

Oh well...not a stellar day today. Unfortunately, pain management suffered a little...not do to with the outstanding care Jo-Ann is getting from hospital staff...just due to the nature of the beast. The doctors warned us that pain levels might spike for a short while...and spike they did. Jo-Ann had a bit of a rough morning and afternoon. Percy decided to take the day off (not terribly serious but problematic)...he needs to wake up soon and get back to doing what he does best. Late in the afternoon, the pain became more manageable. Jo-Ann's colour improved...her energy came back...but through it all she never lost her sense of humour or good spirits. Hopefully tomorrow will be a better day. When I left she was comfortable and eating a healthy supper.

Saturday, *March 23, 2013*

A lousy day…an as yet unknown complication has arisen. Jo-Ann had a terrible night (last night)…awoken in the middle of it due to terrific pain. Doctor saw her this morning and took her off food and liquids…back on the IV. She was sent down for a CTScan in the afternoon. We are still awaiting the results. They increased her pain medication which has helped somewhat…but she hates the side effects (she gets a bit wonky). She was finally able to sleep heavily for about 45 minutes just before I left (which is good news). The pain was still at a high level when I left, but somewhat under control. All we can do now is wait. She is receiving terrific care (the staff has been terrific). Keep your fingers, toes, and eyes crossed. Percy is still being a bit stubborn…not yet fully on the job. Hopefully we'll have good news from the doctor tomorrow.

Sunday, *March 24, 2013*

Wow…what a relief today…arrived at the hospital this AM and saw my cutie with a big smile on her face…all rosy cheeked and everything. The problem had been a collection of seroma between the abdominal muscles and the skin. Seroma is a fluid that the body produces as a mechanism to fill any empty spaces left in the body after some surgeries. It is usually absorbed back into the body after healing commences. Unfortunately, while it collects it can augment pain. The medical staff had decided that since Jo-Ann was doing so well the first two days after surgery, they would wean her off of her pain medication sooner than planned. This reduction of pain medication plus the collection to seroma led to the perfect storm…

excruciating pain. The solution was to re-ramp up the pain medication. This provided the necessary relief to allow Jo-Ann to relax and sleep leading to the reduction and reabsorption of seroma fluid. Needless to say, we will continue the pain medication as long as required. Jo-Ann is many times better than she was yesterday…the healing can resume. There was one blessing in this whole episode…the CTScan results indicated that the surgery was completely successful…everything was as it should be. Oh yes, after the alleviation of the pain and stress, Percy came to life and is pooping away merrily…doing the job he was born to do. Jo-Ann was amazing through all this. She was more worried about me and how I was doing (typical)!. She sends her love to all of you and appreciates the messages, thoughts, and prayers. She actually apologized to me for giving us a scare. I left her this evening with a smile on her face looking forward to tomorrow.

Monday, *March 25, 2013*

Jo-Ann and Percy are home…I am content!

We're Back – *March 28, 2013*

Hello Everyone,

Firstly, I would like to thank you all for your love and support. I felt each and every one of you with me.

For the first time since the surgery I am able to sit up at the computer for a short while. I wanted to ensure that my first post was sent out as soon as it was possible for me.

Considering what has occurred I am doing as well as possible. I have a home care nurse that comes each day to attend to my wound care. They are also going to send me an ET nurse (specialist who works with stomas). I'm still on morphine and another pain killer and for the most part the pain management is working. So, if some of this posting doesn't make sense, I can blame it on the meds.

Percy underwent major work, he was also re-seated. This has caused a great deal of trauma for him. He's still swollen, flush with fever and he is not online yet. By this I mean the poor little fella has been unable to produce a substantial poop for 9 days now. This is starting to be a bit rough on us, but with stool softeners we do hope that Percy will wake up soon. I think he's simply traumatized by the whole situation.

Unfortunately, I have had to endure a number of complications that will be cleared up soon. I ended up with a bladder infection, and infection in the wound while in hospital. I was put on antibiotics and as a result of the medication I am now enjoying a full blown case of thrush. I do hope that all of this will calm down within the next few days.

My spirits are high, I'm not a Ms. Grumpy Pants yet, hope I can keep this up. The body is another story entirely, I am waiting for the days where I can say, "Hmm...I'm feeling better with each passing day".

I do hope you appreciated Mark's (Hubby) efforts to keep you as up to date as possible. After spending full days in hospital with me, dealing with all the things an advocate must deal with, he then would come home and write the updates.

Once again thank you everyone. I will do my best to send an update post as often as is possible for me. Percy & I miss you all.

Jo-Ann L. Tremblay
Ostomate
"Every one you meet has a story to tell."

Thar She Blows – *April 4, 2013*

The healing journey is an interesting dance. It's a one step at a time forward, with a leap or a bound thrown in for good measure. Then there's the sideways stomp and the occasional backslide. Yet, progress is made in this freestyle dance.

Percy has had a challenging time of it. We underwent surgery March 19th and it wasn't till March 29th, that Percy started to wake up. Poor little stoma was traumatized from the procedures, he had simply shut down. Little Percy pooper was pooped out. He has since slowly but surely woken up and is returning to a healthy pungent self, and is once again starting to immerse himself in his liquidation business. What a pooper trooper!

I continue to make the necessary healing strides with the help of my caregiver and husband Mark, my Health Care Nurse, and my cheerleading friends and family. Thanks for joining in the dance with me everyone.

I'm still on a cocktail of pain management drugs that make my brain wonky, 2 forms of antibiotics, and few more prescriptions thrown in. Mentioning pain management drugs, Percy is looking forward to posting the next blog, not sure what he'll come up with, but I'm expecting that I'll be at the butt end of his potty humour.

The 24 hours leading up to Wednesday, April 3rd were quite tense for me. That was the date 21 of my total 31 surgical staples were scheduled to be removed. Now, I'm not normally a nervous nellie, but in my rather more distant past when surgical stitches were removed the whole incision opened up and came fully apart. A traumatic experience to say the least.

And so, the night of April 2nd the words, "Thar She Blows", screamed throughout a dream filled night. I woke up in the morning with it still on my mind as I awaited for my Health Care Nurse to arrive. I had informed her of my concerns the day before, and so, when she arrived she was aware and considerate. She settled into her task and one by one removed the staples. I'm glad to say, it all went well, the incision did not open up, and there was no, "Thar She Blows". I am relieved this stage of the healing journey is behind me, and I'm looking forward to the day when I'm well enough to dream, "Thar She goes".

Jo-Ann L. Tremblay
Ostomate
"Everyone you meet has a story to tell."

A Bedtime Story – *April 9, 2013*

Jo-Ann and I continue our healing journey and every day there seems to be challenges and triumphs. For the past few days Jo-Ann has had difficulty in finding a pain free sleeping position, as she weans down from her pain management medication. This has been rather disconcerting to say the least. Never ones' to be in a state of frustration for too long, Jo-Ann and I are facing the challenge by reaching into our bag of tricks, and coming up with a resourceful solution.

Ongoing since I was created July 21, 2011, Jo-Ann has from time to time had difficulty staying asleep all night. We're incontinent, and so, there are nights when I'm active and we have to do our maintenance. No matter what time it is, it's not always easy to go right back to sleep.

No use tossing, turning, getting frustrated nor fretting, because sometimes we meditate, we pray, we count sheep, and so on. These don't work every time though, Jo-Ann isn't always sure when I'm finished my activities. I've decided these nights are not so bad really, that's because Jo-Ann will tell me a bedtime story. She fills her head with images and stretches her imagination. Her stories are usually quite funny, and they have a moral to each of them. In the quiet of the night when everyone is asleep, together we weave the fabric of imagination and walk through the misty night tracks, to arrive at the Runs River in the land of Flange. On some of our visits we dance with Prince Colon. On other nights we join Lady Catheter of Tube, for some titillating conversations.

So if you have one of those nights, you know the one's where you just have to go with the flow, here's one of Jo-Ann's bedtime stories to entertain you, and help you fall asleep.

The Duke Of Flange

Long ago there lived the Duke of Flange, who was responsible for overseeing the Department of Incontinence Difficulties. Every day the Duke would say, *"If only we could control the flow of the Runs River"*. But for a long time there was no control.

Then came the day of the great Esprit de Corps Festival . The harvest was in and many came from all over to feast and celebrate. As each attempted to cross the Runs River, the raging torrent bubbled and boiled, making the crossing treacherous indeed. To the dismay of the Duke of Flange most were turning back, it was not safe.

The Duke quickly called together the Privy Council to once and for all find a way to control the Runs River. Sir Paper of Toilet, Lady Irritable of Bowel, Prince Colon, Queen Urethra, and King Convexity were the first to arrive, followed by many others. They discussed, considered, and discussed the matter some more, no solutions came to mind.

Then in their darkest moments of dismay, someone quietly entered. *"My name is Percy, I am but a humble stoma. We have long awaited our Festival and our invited guests to arrive"*, he shouted. *"I have the solution"*, he proclaimed. Everyone went silent and turned to hear what the humble stoma had to say.

"The Runs River has a mighty flow. This flow reminds us of the nutrients of the land that we need in order to stay healthy and prosperous. There are no blockages. As the River twists through the narrows it provides us with all that is good. Let us not block the movement, let us not stem the flow. Instead, let us wait it out. Have patience, the Runs River does not always flow so wild. After the time of the great torrent, the Runs River always returns to normal. It is then that we will send out the messengers and invite all to join in our Festival, and we will feast as we celebrate".

Everyone was silent, no sound was made. It was then that the Duke of Flange embraced and encircled Percy the humble stoma and shouted, *"Your words are wise. We will wait out the great torrent, and then all will be well."* King Convexity and Queen Urethra stepped forward and declared, *"From this day forward you will be addressed as and will hold all of the titles of; Percy Stoma – Eol. Of Poopology. Thank you for your great service".* Everyone cheered.

I do hope you enjoyed one of our bedtime story adventures, the moral of this story is; We can't control everything, but we can take control. We are incontinent that is our challenge. Humour, creativity and some resourcefulness is our victory.

Percy Stoma
Eol. Poopology
"Better With A Bag Than In A Bag"

Percy Has Star Quality – *April 22, 2013*

During our recovery Percy (Stoma), has become the star of the show, or, maybe he's just seeing stars. Let's step back and find out how this all came about.

Biography

Jo-Ann L. Tremblay on Percy

Created in Ottawa on 21 July 2011 Percy started his existence by being a life saver, right from the get go. His first of many public presentations was to the resident ET (Enterostomal Therapy) Nurse, within a few days of creation at hospital. He returned to Orleans, Canada later that month and with an unsnap of his bag he continued to perform presentations for a multitude of audiences that included; community ET Nurses, Home Care Nurses and Doctors, which in his opinion made him an overnight success.

Percy settled down to the life of a stoma; pooping, passing wind, writing and posting blogs, at the same time broadening his activities as a model for custom designed haute pooture underwear that accommodate stomas and their bags, while providing abdominal support.

Percy's reputation grew steadily, helped by earning an Eol. of Poopology, (Eol. **E**xperience **O**f **L**ife), given to celebrate Jo-Ann's recovery from major illness, and a 2nd chance at life.

2012 saw continued recovery and the publication of a book based on his life and adventures, for which he also modelled for the oil paining, *"Percy A Self-Portrait"*, that graces the front cover of, *"Better With A Bag Than In A Bag"*.

Public presentations followed as he was uplifted by a honey dew mellon sized parastomal hernia, these included nurses, ET Nurses, specialists, and physicians . A 2nd collaboration with his surgeon who originally created him, resulted in major surgery March 2013, a surgery performed with the intent of designing an internal environment conducive for a higher quality of life.

He has now re-united with Home Care Nurses on a daily basis for wound care, visited the hospital emergency for a post surgery concern, and was recently measured and fitted for a customized abdominal hernia belt.

His most ambitious work is yet to come, a full recovery without a parastomal hernia re-occurrence.

Now, I must admit Percy has been enduringly popular as he removes his bag and bares himself without self-consciousness during his private and public medical presentations. He is quite proud of his new more svelte profile, much to my discomfort, embarrassment and desire for privacy.

Most of us feel our dignity is compromised when due to medical issues we are required to expose and share our body and/or life parts that we would much rather keep private. Understandable and normal I feel. Embarrassment aside, no matter the body or life part that is potentially ill, injured, in recovery, or should have regular check ups, it's important that we indulge in medical presentations and scrutiny.

The jury is still out as to whether Percy is the star of the show, or, he's just seeing stars. I regard his performances as private and public benefit presentations that are an advantage to both of us to receive from. Next time you have to bare and share part of yourself you would rather not make public (like during a colonoscopy for example), just think of it as a command benefit performance from which you will be glad that you attended, even if it struck an emotional chord.

Jo-Ann L. Tremblay
Ostomate
"Everyone you meet has a story to tell."

Thank You, Thank You, A Thousand Times Thank You – *May 3, 2013*

Woo hoo, skippy skippy, and a resounding poopalicious cheer from Percy. Thursday, May 2, 2013, Percy and I reached a milestone, our Home Care Nurse signed us off. For the past 5 weeks she visited us once a day, then every second day, and finally in the last two weeks every third day, gently tending to our surgery wound care. She arrived with a smile, a big hello, and then settled down to inspect our surgical wound and administer her healing magic. Always the professional with that personal touch.

Now as Percy says, *"poopologically speaking we should be ecstatic"*, yet, I find myself feeling strangely adrift. I have taken the last couple of days to explore this odd feeling and have realized; when we are vulnerable, injured, in pain, and require expertise beyond ourselves, we place a great deal of confidence in those folks who are there to help us. They are in our lives during our weak time, and we look forward to them being there with us. We trust they have the know how to keep us safe, as they encourage us along our healing journey. They are our cheerleaders encouraging us along the way.

Then, the day comes when we don't need them anymore. This bond we had established, this healing team that scored so many goals, is now disbanded.......

Of course it's time to move on, the healing is underway and full recovery is the ultimate goal. As humans we need to live with, for, and by one another. So thank you to all the health care professionals for your healing magic, and for being the best cheerleaders a patient can hope for.

My musings brought me to another member of the healing team. Our personal caregiver, Mark, my husband. I'm so fortunate to have a caregiver, and I encourage everyone to think about helping others in their time of need, if for no other reason than you never know when you may need that shoulder to lean on.

And so, as I reminisce the past few years that included my illness, near death, 2 major surgeries, recovery that has now taken up years of our lives, and through all of it we were together, a team, and we've fought the good fight. In celebration of Mark, and for all the caregivers of the world, I have written *"Ode To My Caregiver"*. Your love, care, concern and commitment, is one of the greatest gifts you will ever give. Thank you.

Ode To My Caregiver
Eyes glazed over and lying on my back,
Through the darkness I gaze up to you;
Conspiring together to keep me on track.
The things you want to affect are mine too,
We blend our roles as the 1000 mile healing journey begins,
Terrified, filled with fear and pain,
Your humanity glowing shines through.

Fighting for my body to take control, and keeping my mind sane,
Cold and dark when we set out, as my body strength dims,
Until I think the decent into the dark will never cease,
I look up to you as our combined strength binds.

Your steady hands and feet are mine,
Through the cloud of pain I gaze up to you.

Hard at work you are, so I may dine,
With gentle smiles you tenderly help me feel rosy blue,
Your humanity glowing shines through.

Strong laden shoulders lift the burdens from me,
Each day my healing journey continues to haste;
Committed to your charge you minister to,
With patience and dedication to set healing more;
At the end of the dying day, how can I your patient but adore,
Wrapped in the warmth of your care I feel safe.

The mood is much brighter as the days pass,
With a swell of joy and admiration I gaze up to you.
So many times through the uncertainty we found ourselves
thrash,
Yet, we also found our pace forward steady and true,
Your humanity glowing shines through.

Close bosom-friend of the healing journey,
Joining me in the dance, 2 steps forward, a slide to the side,
Then, 1 step backward, followed by 2 more forward, now let's
hurry.
Always hand in hand dear caregiver we are,
As we look to the end of our journey now not so far,
Thank you, thank you, a thousand times thank you.

Jo-Ann L. Tremblay

Triumph Of The Human Spirit – Lizzie's Story – *May 16, 2013*

This, the age of communication provides us with the everyday opportunities to connect with our community of humanity, globally. We exchange our thoughts and messages beyond boundaries faster and farther than our ancestors before us.

From the far reaches of our World, we journey out through the global web to touch and be touched with our expressions and interactions. We communicate our conscious ideas with the intent someone(s), somewhere, will read and interpret our messages in ways that are significant to them.

Since Percy's creation, I have made the commitment to support ostomy awareness for the benefit of people currently affected, and to those who may be affected by bowel disease in the future. Regardless of age, gender or race, there are legions of people the world over with bowel diseases, colorectal cancer and ostomates, who are intimately connected with family, caregivers/advocates and medical professionals. Oh by the way, Percy says he's definitely along for the joy ride, too.

I believe no matter our condition in life, we all have the potential courage even when we are in pain or experiencing adversity, to create and live a full and joyous quality of life, in spite of it ALL.

I chose to create, "THE OSTOMY FACTOR" blog using the global communication web as a platform to share. My hope is to engage the passion and emotion in all of us to embrace our individual and collective power, no matter who we are, where we are, and no matter our life circumstances.

This week I received an email from an amazing woman who lives in Zimbabwe, Africa. She has a story to tell, and has graciously allowed me to share it with you. Although this is a fellow ostomates' life story, it is a story for everyone. She inspires me, and in the spirit of connecting with our community of humanity for the purpose of touching and being touched, this is her story, in her own words.

Lizzie's Story

Dear Jo-Ann

I got sick at the age of 12, had stomach pains, constant diarrhea, was given wrong treatment which contributed to worsening my health, lost weight and was even at some point told that I had AIDS. I was always in and out of hospital, dropped out of school, was operated on at the age of 20 by one of the doctors who told me I had ulcerative colitis, and I wished I had gotten in contact with him years back.

I got my stoma, and at first it was a huge shock, I said to myself, "my life would never be better and normal again". I had no idea what a stoma was, how to clean or how it would work. I did not have any idea at all. After the operation my health started getting better, started gaining weight, no pains, it was an amazing miracle, indeed.

2006 I was using plastic bags on my stoma, I didn't know that there were ostomy appliances I could use. Then early 2007 I got in contact with ILCO Sweden, then they started sending ostomy appliances. I thought I was the only person in Zim-

*babwe who had an ostomy, but was amazed with the re-
sponse I got from a newspaper article I wrote.*

*From the ostomy appliances I got from Sweden I started shar-
ing them with other ostomy patients here in Zimbabwe. 2011 I
had reached over 300 patients, had formed 6 support groups
in 6 provinces. Got registered as an organization, and getting
more appliances from Sweden, and other well wishing ostomy
organizations and companies around the world.*

*Have since got assistance from Sweden also in training on
ostomy, and use of appliances. Traveled to Sweden with my
sister who is helping me. My family has been a huge pillar of
support to me and the program.*

*Most of the ostomy patients have no information at all about
what a stoma is and how to clean. We are the only organization in Zimbabwe that is operating assisting ostomates, and
that has information on ostomy, some of the activities we do
include:*

- *support groups*

- *counselling*

- *trainings on ostomy care, to ostomates, caregivers,
  nurses, etc.*

- *information dissemination on ostomy*

- *psycho-social support*

- *spiritual support*

- *visits before and after operation in hospitals, at home
  and telephone*

- *income generating programs*

Yes, we are still getting assistance from Sweden, they collect appliances from other ostomates in their country who do not need them anymore and have them in supply, from hospitals and other well wishers, and they send them to us. They have been very helpful and we are grateful for the support that they are giving us. Currently there are no companies producing the ostomy appliances locally.

Oh and I forgot to mention, my stoma is for life, and I got married in 2010, and gave birth to a healthy baby boy in 2011. My husband accepted me the way I am with my stoma, and all four of us, my husband, son, stoma and I, we are living a happy life. Life couldn't be better than this.

Thank you

Lizzie
Country Coordinator
Ileostomy and colostomy Zimbabwe Trust
ILCO ZIM TRUST

"Everyone you meet has a story to tell."

Fellowship Of The Bag – *June 5, 2013*

"To Know the Road Ahead...Ask Those Coming Back"- Chinese Proverb

In the beginning when I was created, Jo-Ann and I felt very much in isolation. We lamented as we experienced a profound lack of fellowship in that present time, and extending into our future. Beyond the pain Jo-Ann felt throughout her body as she recovered from the disease that preceded my creation and my creation surgery itself, I sensed another pain inside. We were alone, an isolated island stranded in a void of empty space. We were grasping for threads of knowledge, understanding, and a sense of community.

Everyone we knew eliminated in the way nature designed them to. We were different now, what nature intended no longer existed for us. I am destined to have a bag over me, the buck stops here. At that time, we felt we were sailors in the midst of a shipwreck.

I did my best to keep us moving, (so to speak), being as adventurous and humorous as I could be, considering it was the early days. We had many ostomy questions that no one in our circle of family nor friends could answer. We were experiencing physical/emotional issues and feelings, that no one could relate to.

We had wonderful friends, family, and a legion of medical experts surrounding us who were concerned. So many in the most precious of ways, reached out and reacted from their perception that we were in distress, and so, in need of them. They extended loving and caring words and gestures stemming from their concern for our well-being. Others pitied us, and still others just didn't know what to say or do. We thank all of them, and hold them dear in Jo-Ann's heart.

But, for us something was missing. We were not normal anymore, we were on the journey to a new normal. There were no road maps, nor fellow ostomate travellers on the path. As we reached out to those around us, we still felt in need. We were rich in sympathy from others, we were surrounded by care and concern, yet, we felt alone on the road.

Step by step, Jo-Ann began to take control of my ostomy care. Then, one day she noticed a grapefruit sized bulge under me. What was it? What was wrong with me? We were frightened of what it might be! Jo-Ann started making phone calls to the surgeon, family doctor, and home care nurses. Although we did not feel physically different from the day before, we were terribly frightened as to what the bulge might mean. Desperate for some understanding, Jo-Ann searched the internet and found the phone number of our regions' United Ostomy Association of Canada, (UOAC) – support group. The support groups have volunteers who are available to answer ostomy questions.

A gentleman called us back within an hour and helped put Jo-Ann's mind at ease. This was our introduction to the cool dudes and dudettes of the UOAC. This volunteer-run charitable organization is dedicated to helping all persons, including families and caregivers, who are affected by ostomy surgery. We have learned so much from our connection with them, and the camaraderie is priceless. There are United Ostomy Associations worldwide.

It was at this time we found what we were missing, the reason why we felt so adrift, we needed empathy!

No matter your situation in life, whether you have a bowel disease, ride a motor cycle, are going through a divorce, you are an entrepreneur, battling cancer, or whatever life issue or situation is yours to experience, there are associations in your region. Everyone needs to know there are others out there with the ability to mutually experience the thoughts, emotions and direct experiences, as you. We are not alone. We are not an island. We are not adrift. In fact, all of us are surrounded by people who are just like us. These are people who understand what we are going through, because they have gone through it themselves. Empathy is a treasure we can all discover. As a community of humanity, we are in fact part of a far richer reality.

Percy Stoma
Eol. Poopology
"Better With A Bag Than In A Bag"

This post was written due to memories sparked by an inspirational email sent to us by Larry in Jersey City, USA. Following is an excerpt from his email:

EMPATHY
Empathy differs from sympathy. People in the medical, nursing and healing professions can offer sympathy for a patient's disease or defect and the need for an ostomy.
The offering of empathy, though, can be done only by ostomates; only they have the unique understanding derived from experiencing a similar situation.
Without even a word, the sight of a vigorous individual with an inconspicuous ostomy is testimony to the acceptability of a stoma.
Beyond the reassuring appearance comes the shared concerns and triumphs, solutions to problems, answers to questions.

This exchange makes easy the rehabilitation of new
ostomates and is a source of enormous pleasure to
those who are reaching out to a fellow human being.
"To Know The Road Ahead . . Ask Those Coming Back!"

The Ostomy Alliance
ostomyvisitor@aol.com

One Day, One Moment, One Breathe At A Time – *July 9, 2013*

The lazy, hazy days of our Canadian summer are in full swing, and its time for many of us to spend as much time outside with friends and family as we can possibly pack in. Goodness knows it's such a short season for us who live north of the 49th latitudinal parallel.

We have just arrived back home from enjoying a week long road trip to attend eldest daughter Beth's wedding, then visiting a dear friend of 40 years, finishing with a visit with our grand daughter Charlie.

Percy (stoma) was as polite as he could possibly be. He would like me to tell you he's proud to say, we had to make only 1 emergency stop. He was quite excited after eating lunch on the road, and had a raging oops moment. All in all, Percy handled things in the way that Percy does. Over excited on some occasions causing me issues, and then too quiet on other occasions causing some issues. There is no doubt Percy gives me endless reasons for laughing at myself and life.

How exquisite, how amazing it is to have a 2nd chance at life. From the brink of death, to, hugging Beth, seeing her marry and start a new life with her wonderful Chris, and then having the opportunity to caress Charlie and smell her baby fresh skin. It's the icing on the cake, the cherry on top!

I've always maintained my love of life whether it was my first go at it, and now at my 2nd round, and yet, there are challenging realities I've come to realize. There is only so much we can do. At times we make mistakes, and at other times we make bad choices. For many of us there will be a point in our lives when we face losing it all, it tears at us, and we won't go down without a good fight. Everyone we meet has their story, and ostomates are no exception.

As I was sitting in the car during the last leg of our road trip monitory my little buddy Percy for any activity as he is wont to do at some of the most inconvenient of times, my mind wandered back to 2008, and then to my painful recovery journey during the summer of 2011.

Following is an excerpt from, *"Better With a Bag Than In a Bag"*, discussing one of my strategies for living in awareness during the best of times, and the hardest of times.

Excerpt: In 2008, when my illness and pain had become chronic, there were times when I was only able to take life one day at a time. Through the years that followed, I was eventually reduced to coping with my body and life one moment at a time. During these times, I often found myself searching, trying to find any reason, any excuse, to have a positive attitude, a positive outlook. I, of course could find many. I am very fortunate to be blessed in so many ways. But as time advanced along with the illness, I realized that I could not go forward on positive thoughts alone. In fact, I realized that I was not being totally honest with myself in thinking I was being positive while knowing in my heart that I was downright miserable. My mind was in a push-me-pull-me mode. I endured the physical pain as I was drowning in an emotional quagmire. I was sick, angry, and fighting for my quality of life.

As the illness progressed, I arrived at the realization that I was taking life one breath at a time now. It was becoming more and more challenging to remain honestly positive so I decided there must be another way. I could try to talk myself into "positive thinking" until I was blue in the face, but in reality there came the understanding that this approach, this life tool, was not working for me anymore. It was not the appropriate tool for this circumstance. It was not real. It was a mask. It was dishonest. It was downright denial. I needed to step down into the depths of my current reality with eyes wide open. Be truthful with myself. I had to look the monster of my illness and my predicament in the eye, with full awareness.

Aha! Awareness. That's the ticket! I began to insert awareness as a coping tool, rather than positive thinking more often than not. In my attempts to simply be aware in the very breaths I took. I used this tool to help develop a deeper understanding of my individuality and the many aspects of myself, my illness, and the life all around me. With full awareness focused and interwoven into each breath, I eventually became sensitive to the truths I was operating from, those I was expressing, and the true realities of my situation. It was honesty, not a fantasy in all its wonder and all of its ugliness. A value-added bonus to this approach was an immersion into the fullness of breath. With every inhale and exhale I realized that time expanded, on occasion to the place of forever. I was beyond positive thinking and had arrived at a place where I realized that any one of us can die at any time. It could be today, it could be tomorrow, or in twenty years from now – who really knows? The only thing that is true is that the "now", the "present", is the reality that exists. It is up to us to put as much into and receive as much as possible from that breath, that moment, that day. I was hurting in all ways possible, so it was hard to see a positive future, but it was easy to immerse into my breath and explore the depths, wonders, and potentials a breath can hold. Like a string of pearls, my string of breaths encircled me with the hope and the strength that life – at least for the moment – continued.

I live in awareness because I could die today, tomorrow, or in twenty years from now. I really don't know. Awareness as a tool works for all times, circumstances and situations during the course of a lifetime. Positive thinking is a great tool, one that is appropriate when we are working hard and anticipating a successful outcome. Positive thinking is a tool of great usefulness, but it is not the only tool in our personal and professional toolbox.

Sitting on my patio on those warm summer days during my recovery. I found myself looking back, and looking forward. Awareness is a valuable tool I will use quite regularly and continue to hone as my life continues to unfold.

Jo-Ann L. Tremblay
Ostomate
"Everyone you meet has a story to tell."

Percy & I Are Thrilled – *July 29, 2013*

"Better With A Bag Than In A Bag" is #10 on the Indie Author Land top #10 Chart for summer reads. To see the chart,
go to: bit.ly/IndieTopTen23. You can read the Indie Author
Land interview at to http:/bit.ly/IndieAL46.

Enjoy, thank you.

Jo-Ann L. Tremblay & Percy Stoma

When Things Go Bump In The Night –
August 12, 2013

My grandmother was born in 1895. Filled with sage advice, she lived just over 100 years. I was blessed with knowing her, well into my adult life. When in her 90's, Mémère got up sometime during the night for a glass of water. Filling her glass, she then stood straight up, lifted the glass to her lips, and with head tilted back she took a sip of water. It was at this time she lost her balance, fell backwards, hit the floor and broke her back. Being the resilient and amazing woman she was, in time she healed, and went on with her life armed with another life lesson learned.

During one of our many visits she stated, *"If you get up during the night, be cautious. You'll notice when a dog or your cat wakes up from a sleep, they take their time. They stretch this way, and then that way before they walk away. That's natures' wisdom in action, Jo-Ann. Take your time getting out of bed and moving. We're not fully coordinated in body and mind when just waking from a deep sleep."*

Well, I guess I forgot about that particular wisdom. It was early morning a few weeks ago, at about 4:00 a.m., when my enigmatic and spirited Percy decided to overact. Cozy in my bed and through the fog of a forgotten dream, I suddenly became aware of number two of the final act of digestion quickly filling Percy's bag.

A far cry from graceful I bounded out of bed with lights off. In our sleeping house I moved at lightening speed toward the bathroom. As I reached what I guessed was the bathroom doorway, my balance became completely out of control. I lost myself somewhere in the middle of the best or the worse out-come in that split second. You know, when we are free falling and time expands giving us the opportunity to experience lightness, dread and panic, as we hang somewhere in be-tween dimensions of time and space. *"Will I be okay, or am I heading for a crash, and what can I do about it?!?"*

My automatic response in place, I fling my right hand and arm out to grab the doorframe. At the very extension of my skin I feel the feather touch of the frame. Damn, I missed and now I'm heading into the door frame face and full Percy frontal, accident bound.

In the following instant I decided to do what I thought quite clever of me; I torqued my body counterclockwise in midair, and crashed my right hip into the doorframe, instead. With an explosion of pain on impact, I then gathered my wits about me, and limped into the bathroom.

Later that morning the pain in my hip was so intense, it was off to the "Urgent Care Clinic", I headed.

"You're fortunate, no bone fracture. You have a severe deep bruising and it's going to hurt like stink for about 2 weeks. I could prescribe pain killers", stated the Doctor.

"Nope, I've had enough of that stuff since my most recent surgery in the spring. I can handle it", said I.

"Well, my best advice to you", continued the Doctor, *"is like the old joke: A guy goes to the Doctor. The Doctor asks how he can help him. The guys says, Doc it hurts when I do this. And, the Doctor says, then don't do it"*.

"Thanks Doc", I said as I departed the clinic, and proceeded to limp my way to the car. I crawled into the drivers seat and headed home.

Prepared for right hip pain for a fortnight, I was surprised when 6 days later an intense pain, left of my spine settled in and started to expand across my lower back, left hip and down my thigh. *"Oh great, I must have pulled a muscle during my ever so clever torque"*, I thought.

For a couple of weeks following, I had good and then not-so-good days. As predicted, within 2 weeks the right hip got better and better, finally it's as good as any hip my age can feel.

Unfortunately, my left lower back, hip and leg seemed to get progressively worse. Finally, a week ago I found myself unable to stand up from a sitting position. The pain in my back was excruciating and I was literally stuck in the lounge chair.

Once again, it's off to the Urgent Care Clinic, with Percy and I feeling like crap.

"Well, there's been more damage than originally thought. You have a disk injury. I'm prescribing an anti-inflammatory and pain killer, and here's a prescription for physio therapy. It will hurt like stink for another 4 weeks", said my sympathetic Doctor.

Now, off to physio therapy, in addition to the disk injury, upon further examination it is found out that my sacrum , (the large, triangular bone at the base of the spine and at the upper and back part of the pelvic cavity, that is inserted like a wedge between the two hip bones, the upper connects with the last lumbar vertebra, and bottom part to the tailbone), is awkwardly out of alignment.

Percy and I are now attending our physio appointments 3 times a week. We're responding well to the medication, and we're looking forward to being as good as new in a few weeks.

Upon hearing about our misadventure, my friend and fellow ostomate Carol reminded me, *"It's frustrating how ostomies complicate even the simplest thing at times, even when it isn't quite the ostomy doing anything".*

Okay, Percy you're off the hook, you're no longer in the poop house.

The moral of this sharing is: To avoid the misadventures of things going bump in the night, remember our dogs and cats, with or without a stoma and at any age, take time to orientate your mind and wake your body before bounding out of bed!

Jo-Ann L. Tremblay
Ostomate
"Everyone you meet has a story to tell."

The Case Of The Raging Toilet – *September 4, 2013*

An ostomates life can seem a bit silly at times, especially when we have to leave treasures all over our community. Percy and I went out to run a number of errands the other morning. Percy (my enigmatic spirited stoma), decided to overact as I drove the car to the Passport Office. As we traveled each kilometre after another, well, what can I say, instead of our cup runneth over, our bag was just about there and it seemed to me, we hit every red light cosmically possible.

Finally we arrived at our destination with not more than a moment to spare. First stop, was to the bathroom to take care of Percy's business, before we addressed my business. Up one hall, nope no bathroom, down another hall, nope no bathroom. With frankly no time left, I found a commissionaire, who gave me directions. "Oh, for Pete's sake, I must have passed it at least twice", I thought.

With a great deal of relief I dealt with Percy, and to make life easy and efficient for me, I simply went into my "Percy's spare equipment stash", that I keep in my purse for a fresh bag, and deposited Percy's old treasure bag well packaged into the washroom trashcan.

With everything in order it was now time to go back down the hall to the Passport office. When this task was completed it was time to head off to the grocery store. As the life of an ostomate would have it, Percy once again thought this was quite exciting, as I suddenly became aware of number two of the final act of digestion quickly filling Percy's bag.

Upon arriving at the grocery store, it was off to the washroom, we headed. I changed once again to a new bag, and deposited Percy's not so old treasure bag in the trashcan.

Groceries purchased, it was off to our final stop – the Pharmacy. Wouldn't you know it, Percy wasn't finished yet, silly little pooper. Well, history had to repeat itself. It was straight home from there, and I wearily stepped through the door. From the moment I entered all was quiet, nothing was moving, not even a mouse.

Figuring that with 1 bag, 2 bags, 3 bags I had already filled and almost overflowed, I thought all would be quiet and uneventful for the evening. Hmm....best laid plans of mice and men. Before I go on with the story, know that the whole ordeal has worked out well, and my husband has seen his Physician. Now back to the case of raging toilet.

Our day had not ended, at 11:30 p.m. it was off to the Emergency Care Unit of our local hospital for a medical issue for my husband Mark. By 1:00 a.m., pungent Percy, kicked into high gear yet again. The toilet facility was adjacent to Mark's room. I went in to deal with Percy, all went well, until I flushed the toilet.

Well, a tornadic fury began, then a counterclockwise rotation of speed and noise I have never witnessed before in the water closet raged and would not stop. Around, around and around, like a tempest in a tea pot it raged. Then as I danced about jiggling the toilet handle in an attempt to stop the torrent, a small geyser erupted in the middle of the rotation, and a fine spray of water filled the air above the toilet, and a mist began to fill the area.

It was at this time I escaped the washroom as a nurse heard the roar of the toilet, and came over to the door to peer in with me. No sooner had he witnessed the raging toilet, it began to slow down and it eventually stopped. It had stopped as mysteriously as it had started. He then turned to me and said, *"Well, that must have been some log you deposited"*.

Jo-Ann L. Tremblay
Ostomate
"Everyone one you meet has a story to tell."

Did You Hear About The One About... -
September 9, 2013

We're very excited, **"Better With a Bag Than In a Bag"** is being sold by Amazon throughout North America, Europe, and Japan, and is now available with Half.com, BarnesandNoble, and with Alibris. Visit "Better With a Bag Than In a Bag" book page on this blog site to find out more information and to click on the links. As some of you may have not read, the book yet , I thought it might be fun to share several excerpts from the book for your reading enjoyment. Before you start, I just want you to know the book was written during my year long recovery from the lifesaving surgery that created "Percy". If you're interested in laughing, crying, and guffawing, as I hope you do when you read THE OSTOMY FACTOR blog posts, you'll truly enjoy reading the book.

Excerpt from PART 1 – THINGS ARE GOING DOWNHILL

Disturbing TRUTHS!

The following day, lying in bed in a morphine and epidural haze, I am roused when the team walks in. The General Hospital in Ottawa, Canada is a teaching hospital. Therefore, four of the eight-member team of doctors who had worked on me through the surgery the day before came and stood by my bed. With them was a gaggle of resident medical students. A good looking crew they were, and eager to explain to me how bad my situation had been, what had happened, and what amazing medical miracles they had performed..........

I was stunned to say the least. "My descending bowel had multiple perforations?" Things had been very bad with my intestines. Hmm . . . Swiss cheese comes to mind. "Let me get this straight: I had perforations throughout the sigmoid region of the colon......"

And so, eight separate doctors, each with their own special-ized expertise, repaired my body parts. Well, how wonderful of them," I said..........

"Oh, you performed a Hartman's procedure. The sigmoid sec-tion — I know that one. It's the descending colon, right? — of my large bowel. It was removed. Part of my rectal stump was also removed. Oh. I see."

"Wait a minute! You said you had to perform a Hartman's pro-cedure. I have a colostomy. OK, what the heck does all that mean?"...........

Outdoor Plumbing

> "Sigmoid colostomy is a procedure when fecal diversion is required," stated the head of the team. "We have di-verted the fecal stream from the rectum and anus. This was necessary to remove the area of diseased bowel. We removed a section of your descending bowel and rectum. The operation was necessary. Your bowel was diseased and perforated."

"OK. But what happened to me? What's going on? What am I supposed to do now?"

> "We made an incision in your abdomen. We removed the diseased area of the bowel. We had to remove some of your rectal stump. We repaired your damaged ...... And we've made a colostomy."

"Excuse me for not understanding, but what is a colostomy?"

"A colostomy is the end of the colon brought to the surface and stitched to the skin through a small cut in the abdomen. Fecal waste will now pass through the colostomy — it's called a stoma — and it will then be collected in a bag that sticks to the skin with special colostomy equipment. A prosthetic so to speak." And with a satisfied smile, the head guy of this interesting motley crew, simply ended the consultation with, "You have a colostomy."

"Well. My gosh. That explains everything. NOT!"

Brain Freeze

Okay, I'm alive. Check. I have tubes pumping stuff into me and some draining stuff out of me. Check. I'm so filled with drugs I seriously don't know up from down. Check. My body feels numb and weird. Check. I'm pooping into a bag that is attached to my abdomen near my belly button. Check. Oh my gosh. I'm pooping into a bag!

As I press the buzzer for the nurse I am near panic.

"Can I help you," she asks.

"Yes, well, apparently I have a bag attached to me. I'm pooping into the bag. Am I understanding right?"

"Yes, you're understanding."

"OK. So I'm pooping into a bag. How is that working for me? Will I have this for a short while or a long while? Do I have some kind of hole in me? What happens when the bag fills

up? Where do I get bags?" And, the questions kept on float-
ing up through my foggy brain. It was probably a blessing that
my brain was foggy. I think I would have died on the spot from
an anxiety-induced heart attack. Geez, it was all so weird.

> "Mrs. Tremblay, all your questions will be answered in
> due time. You've been through a lot. Just lie back and
> relax. Your next goal is to start working on getting up.
> And then starting to walk. You're on a floor that is not
> used to handling this kind of recovery. All the beds are
> filled on that floor. They're the ones who handle your
> type of situation. Don't worry, though. We're with you
> here and we'll help you through it. Within the next few
> days, the resident ET nurse will be coming to see you for
> a consultation. She'll help you understand your colosto-
> my. She'll instruct you on how to take care of your stoma,
> and so on. Do you need anything else?"

"No, I don't need anything right now, thanks."

Oh my gosh. Those drugs must be really something, I
thought. The hospital is sending an extraterrestrial nurse to
talk with me. Apparently aliens must be the experts in dealing
with my stoma, whatever the heck that is. Not sure why
they're so savvy about poop bags though. Well, I'll just have
to wait and see this amazing being from out there somewhere
who's got all the answers.

It took days before my Florence Night-in-Alien, arrived at my
bedside......

Jo-Ann L. Tremblay
Ostomate
"Everyone you meet has a story to tell"

Goofy Bird Wins The Prize – *October 15, 2013*

"We live on a beautiful planet, our home is a wondrous place filled with drama and visual splendour. An interesting subject will appear, a contrast of light and shadow will become apparent, or a drama will unfold, this is when I focus and snap. A life image and an Earth moment in time is captured, to be enjoyed and relived, over and over again." Artist statement – Jo-Ann L. Tremblay

Percy and I get a real kick out of taking our camera just about everywhere we can, hunting for great photographic shots. Life never ceases to show up, as we delight in snapping away the day. Once again the magic of life showed up last year on Marco Island, Florida, USA.

We were awaiting to board the *"Marco Island Princess"*, for a sunset cruise, and it was a very breezy day. Looking over my shoulder I spotted a Snowy Egret clinging to a railing, holding on for dear life. Her feathers were blowing this way and then that way. A bad feather day would be an understatement. I slowly and carefully walked up to her, camera in my hand and then snapped, we captured her moment.

So as to not stress her any more than she must have been experiencing, I took one more quick photo, and then walked away giving her as wide a berth as possible so that she could do something, anything, to stay upright on the railing and tame her ruffled feathers. Some of us know what that's like first thing in the morning.

I am an author, a painter and I'm also a photographer. Being a member of , "Arteast", in our city, I at times enter my art in juried art exhibitions. This year I decided to enter a photograph, and went about deciding on what photographic pic I would like to exhibit. Interestingly, I was consistently drawn to the pic I call, "Bad Feather Day", and eventually decided on the little Snowy Egret. I did not enter her to win any awards, I entered her because she always makes me smile, chuckle and ponder. And, I am sure she will work her magic on others. Her gift is the gift of humour and steadfastness.

There is another reason why the little one speaks to me, she is a visual metaphor for all of us. Throughout our lives the winds of hardship blow from time to time, threatening to push us over and slam us to the ground. Yet, even with the odds seemingly against us, most of us hang in there, even when it's about hanging on for dear life. All of us who have had a 2nd chance at life know this. Our feathers are ruffled so to speak as we lean in to weather the storms. Our drive to live and get on with getting on with life is intense, even in the most challenging of times.

We don't know if or when the winds will cease. With all the strength and will we have within, we and our support system if we are lucky enough to have one, grasp and cling onto the most solid and steady we can. Being a human is not for wimps! Hurrah to all who choose to live a joyous and the fullest of lives, in spite of it all.

Our little goofy bird's efforts were not in vain, as not only was she accepted for exhibition for the 2013 AJAE (Arteast Juried Art Exhibition), she has been awarded first place in the photography category. From September 29th through November

22nd, 2013, she will give a multitude of people a smile, a chuckle, and maybe just maybe, some inspiration to ponder. Percy and I were delighted to receive our award at the Awards Ceremony. No matter our life situations, we all have hopes and dreams, at times during a lifetime harsh winds blow, like the seemingly delicate Snowy Egret, we're amazingly strong even on our worst bad feather day.

Jo-Ann L. Tremblay
Ostomate
"Everyone you meet has a story to tell."

Oh My...Already?! - *November 13, 2013*

Time certainly flies! One year ago this month Percy and I created, **"THE OSTOMY FACTOR"** blog and published our first posting November 14, 2012, titled, "Chances Are". Our mission is to share the ostomates life, our times, ups, downs, and all arounds with ALL through humour and inspiration.

A lot of water has passed under the bridge, as we experienced the many adventures and misadventures life could throw at us in this past year. During this time, through amazon we indie-published our book, **"Better With A Bag Than In A Bag"**, December 2012. Since then, our real life compelling tale is now available in 8 countries worldwide, (United Kingdom, US, Canada, Germany, France, Italy, Spain, and Japan), and is receiving 5 out of 5 star rated reviews. Folks with ostomies and folks who don't have one have read the book, and the feedback has been more than complimentary. Through humour and inspiration readers are sharing their tears, laughter, stories and human spirit, with Percy, my husband Mark, and I. This has been a true gift for us.

Percy Stoma may have made history by being the first stoma to write blog posts, Percy posted the first stoma to stoma, and, stoma to human blog post December 2012. By this time Percy and I had also painted an oil painting on canvas titled, "Percy A Self Portrait". You can enjoy the art piece every time you look at the cover of, *"Better With A Bag Than In A Bag"*. Stoma's are often referred to as a rose bud. This is due to the fact that the end of the bowel extending externally from the abdomen (stoma), looks like a rose bud.

If you find Percy homely in his actual orientation, flip the book upside down and you will see him as a beautiful rose bud.

What's that? Oh yes, Percy would like you to know the oil painting will be traveling with us, and will be featured at our upcoming speaking engagements. As you can imagine Percy is rather shy and needs to have a bag over his head, and so, Percy is thrilled the painting is up on stage with us providing an opportunity to view him as a representative of one of many stomas around the world who are responsible with keeping their human alive.

Speaking of Percy, the little pungent pooper has quite the sense of humour. As the year moved on and each month progressed my parastomal hernia, a somewhat common complication for ostomates, grew. My abdominal profile which included Percy expanded, we eventually looked about 5 months pregnant on the abdominal left hand side, whilst the right side stayed normal. Not only was this risky health-wise, it also presented a fashion calamity. Percy in his immutable fashion took the opportunity to write the blog post, "Percy Gets A Dress", see the January 28th, 2013 post, and enjoy a good chuckle.

We travelled the winter of 2013, and took the opportunity to visit Kennedy Space Centre in Florida. An inspired Percy embarked on celestial adventures, and he almost became a squished stoma as he was strapped into our seat during the Shuttle launch. See, "Percy Blasts Off", February 22, 2013, blog post.

Interestingly, we as human beings have our gut feelings and we feel "butterflies" in the stomach. Underlying this sensation is an often-overlooked network of neurones lining our guts that is so extensive some scientists have nicknamed it our, "second brain".

A deeper understanding of this mass of neural tissue, filled with important neurotransmitters, is revealing that it does not merely handle digestion or inflict the occasional nervous pang. The little brain in our innards, (no offence to the "little brain" reference is intended Percy), in connection with the big one in our skulls, partly determines our mental state and plays key roles in certain diseases throughout the body.

Although its influence is far-reaching, the second brain is not the seat of conscious thoughts or decision-making. Science tells us that the multitude of neurones in the enteric nervous system enables us to "feel" the inner world of our gut and it's contents. This may explain Percy's compassion when he took on the project of creating and writing the April 9th blog post, "A Bedtime Story". Thanks Percy.

Our blog is reaching out to people all over the world, and many have taken the time to connect back with us. Larry in Jersey City, USA, wrote to us about, "Empathy", which is shared in, "Fellowship of the Bag", June 5th blog post. And, the phenomenal Lizzie who lives in Zimbabwe, Africa, inspired me, and in the spirit of connecting with our community of humanity for the purpose of touching and being touched, I posted, "Triumph Of The Human Spirit – Lizzie's Story", May 16th blog post, in her own words. Thank you Lizzie for your honesty, strength, and commitment to fellow ostomates.

During this past year Percy has settled down to the life of a stoma, pooping, passing wind, writing/posting blogs, and keeping me alive. Percy's reputation has grown steadily, and when we endured the 2nd major surgery in 2 years in March of 2013, Percy and I once again had to battle for our quality of life.

It has been another chapter in an amazing life journey, starting from the time leading up to the 2nd surgery, Percy's DIVA moments while being wheeled into the operating theatre, the zoo, ahem…I mean hospital room and weirdest hospital stay I have ever experienced, our recovery, and our life after life adventures continue. Percy and I are busy writing our next book featuring this amazing journey, we're calling it, **"Another BAG Another DAY"**, and we expect to publish in 2014. Percy and I will keep you posted.

At this time Percy and I would like to express our deepest gratitude to each and every one of you. It is our sincerest hope that you have enjoyed our adventures, learned a few things, had a few chuckles along the way, and have been inspired to take each day as it comes with optimism, in spite of it all. We look forward to continuing the adventures together with you over the next year ahead. Don't forget to leave a comment, we love hearing from you.

All in all, it has been an amazing and at times challenging journey over the past year. I am an ostomate and Percy is a stoma, now we do almost everything I used to do before Percy's creation, and we are able to enjoy everything in life we want to. I have hopes, dreams, and a strong desire to live a joyous and full life, in spite of it all. I was carved into a survivor, Percy keeps me alive, I have a 2nd chance at life – it's the icing on the cake, and the cherry on top!

With Gratitude,
Jo-Ann L. Tremblay
Ostomate,   *"Everyone you meet has a story to tell."*

Percy's Gift – *December 19, 2013*

"You're not a miracle", stated my ear, nose and throat specialist, while I sat in his office."

He wrinkled his nose, viewed my current auditory test results, picked up and viewed my previous test result records, and then looked me in the eye.

"It sometimes happens, we don't always know why", he stated. Then he bowed his head, wrinkled his nose, and continued to view and compare the past and current records. Hmmm..., was the only thought to cross my mind in that moment. Once again, he looked at me straight in the eyes, with what I thought was a strange expression on his face.

Well, that was it, I began to feel weak in the stomach. Little Percy Stoma reacted, and left a little deposit in his bag. My thoughts then raced around in circles. *Oh geez, the other shoe has dropped. Oh no, just when I'm starting to get some of my stamina back. What an odd nose he's got.*

"I'm ordering an MRI, (Magnetic Resonance Imagining), of your ears and head," he went on to say.

Whooo'nelly, was the only focused thought I had left in my head.

"Okay Doctor, what's going on, what are we talking about here, is there something wrong with my ear, my head, what gives?" I managed to get past my lips.

"Oh sorry, yes well, the auditory test results as compared to your previous records are indicating you are actually registering some sounds from your left ear," he finally explained.

At this point I was unable to think or talk yet again for a number of seconds, and I do believe Percy once again made a nervous bag deposit.

This statement is nothing short of a miracle for me, although the Doctor has assured me that I'm not a miracle. You see, I have been profoundly deaf in my left ear since birth!

Hearing loss is the reduced ability to hear sound. Deafness is the complete inability to hear sound. There are many different conditions that lead to partial and total deafness. In my case it's genetics. Several family members have sensorineural deafness. Basically the vestibulocochlear nerve, (auditory vestibular nerve), known as the eighth cranial nerve, transmits sound and equilibrium (balance) information from the inner ear to the brain. I have a nerve disorder, and so, nerve pathways in the brain that normally transmit sound impulses, do not work for me.

At birth and for most of my life the right ear has been high functioning. I've heard very well. But, due to the aging process my right ear hearing has degraded and now functions at a moderate hearing level. About 8 years ago I was fitted with a hearing aid in my right ear only, as it's my only hearing ear, and it has been working as well as can be expected.

"As I mentioned Jo-Ann, this kind of thing happens from time to time, and we often don't always understand why," he stated. "You'll have the MRI appointment within a couple of weeks, this is simply to rule out any abnormal changes, and to give us a clear image of your inner ear," he assured me.

My mind started to race. How amazing, deaf since birth, and now later in life I have gained some ear function. To what extent, time, some hearing device equipment and experimental approaches will reveal. I do not at this time recognize sound from my left ear.

Although there may be any number of reasons for how this has happened, I have my theory, and it goes back 2 years and 5 months ago. I was fighting for my life, as Doctors performed extensive, invasive surgery, and Percy's creation. My disease and the life saving surgery caused almost catastrophic damage to some organs, my bowel system, bladder and so on. Ultimately nerves were also damaged.

I have experienced a myriad of health issues and degraded bodily functions as a direct result of the nerve damage. I have been so fortunate to have had a legion of medical experts from physicians, to, physio therapists working with me these past couple of years. They have worked hard to assist me in gaining as much function and physical feeling to my body parts as possible. Each are incredibly skilled medical professionals with regard to their diagnosis, effective treatment, and good science. I have made great gains, and I am grateful.

But, it's not all up to them, I have a huge part to play in my recovery. In the beginning I decided that one of my healing focuses would be my nerve system, and so, I began to visualize my nerves. I saw them in my mind's eye as vibrant and glowing roots of trees, and branches of bushes.

As I built on this vision I imagined the roots and branches growing and connecting. Within the past few months I have regained full bladder function, and I no longer manifest, "drop foot", just to mention a couple of the gains.

And now, it is becoming apparent that I am also gaining some degree of audio function, that I've never experienced in my life to this point. Frankly, as I flipped my eyes inward to my internal universe, from the beginning I had no idea if my visualization would manifest any results. My primary motivation was simply to increase my sense of control and well-being. My second motivation was to support healing, the regeneration of nerves, and the building of new nerve bridges where required. The mind-body connection has boundaries no doubt, but to what extent? As it turns out, who knows, it's an individual thing. I never imagined that my mind-body journey would bring me to the potential opening of new doors of hearing I've never experienced for more than 5 decades of my life.

The sound world of bird songs, rustling leaves, waves lapping on the beach, the little giggles of grandchildren, and…and… and…, may very well be Percy's gift to me. Sounds I have heard faintly or in theory only, will be music to my ears. The odyssey leading up to Percy's creation, and my ongoing healing process is the gift that keeps giving.

James Gordon, MD, pioneer in Integrative Medicine, states the mind and body are essentially inseparable. "The brain and peripheral nervous system, the endocrine and immune systems, and indeed all the organs of our body and all the emotional responses we have, share a common chemical language and are constantly communicating with one another," states Dr. Gordon.

I gather in my case, my mind didn't distinguish the difference between nerves in my abdomen, spine, nor head. It just went ahead and affected my whole body of nerves. It all began with Percy, and caused me to use my thoughts to positively influence some of my body's physical responses. In the process, I believe, I minimized the negative effects and maximized the healthy, healing aspects of my mind-body connection.

In the spring of 2014, the specialist will outfit me with hearing aids for BOTH ears. I will work with the equipment and the audiologist for a number of months, and who knows how much of the amazing world of sound will open up for me. Thank you Percy.

Percy and I wish everyone a happy, healthy and prosperous 2014.

Jo-Ann L. Tremblay
Ostomate
"Everyone you meet has a story to tell."

Year 3

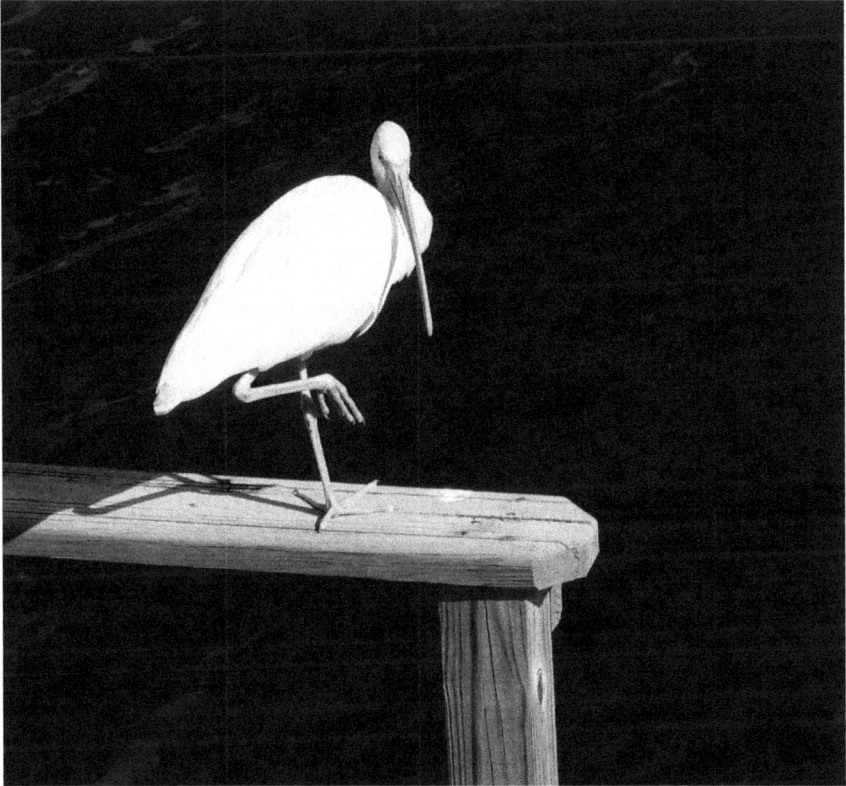

The healing journey is an interesting dance. It's a one step at a time forward, with a leap or a bound thrown in for good measure. Then there's the sideways stomp and the occasional backslide. Yet, progress is made in this freestyle dance.

As Percy Stoma and I dance along the path of life, sometimes we hip-hop feeling close to the ground, there are the break dance days which demands our strength, skill, and balance. On our good days we are able to do pointe work and flow with the precise movements of a ballet, but I must say more often than not, we jitterbug along improvising with each obstacle and challenge.

Living with an ostomy has its ups, downs and all-arounds. It seems as though every week there is something good, something bad, and something humorous about living with Percy Stoma. I have always enjoyed a healthy sense of humour, and I seemed to consistently give myself a daily dose of reasons to laugh at myself and life under my old circumstances. In spite of myself, now that my ostomy has been created, the reasons for laughing at myself and life has increased manyfold.

There are no life journeys I have encountered that are free of issues and obstacles. Life is a challenge, and everyone you meet has a story to tell. I once passed by a shop window, and on display was a finely stitched pillow for sale. It read, "Growing old is not for wimps." Although this is very true, my mind jumped to another thought: "Being human is not for wimps." It gave me a chuckle at the time, and I thought how true it is. Issues, challenges, obstacles, and bumps on the road of life are facts. It is these very life experiences that play a valuable role in our lives. They are the clues, the road signs if you will, that can be used as valuable information when making choices. Road signs are experiences, situations, circumstances, events, happenings, opportunities, and more. We can use them to help us know if we are on track, and they will definitely help point out options. Our personal and professional lives are filled with information we can use that will help us make informed decisions and choices as we do our best to navigate our way to physical and emotional meaningful success.

2014 was a year that I experienced a kaleidoscope of emotions due to the dark and light of life itself. In our lives we experience dark clouds and sunshine, this is the adventure of life unfolding as it will.

Me, Percy and the Tooth Fairy – *January 26, 2014*

As our little planet begins a new orbit around the sun 2014 has begun, it's a new year, marking the start of another path of life to explore. When a new year begins many of us feel stronger and eager to build upon ourselves with aspirations, and inspired resolutions. Best of luck to you all on your path to the future, may it be filled with good health, joy and prosperity.

January 2014 finds Percy, myself and my husband Mark once again in Florida, USA. We've escaped the "arctic vortex", that is holding our Northern home in it's icy grip.

Starting each morning with a walk, Percy and I are captivated by the active life all along the way. We observe great blue herons, american egrets, ibis, little blue herons, and snow egrets. We take the path that brings us to the osprey nest, and observe as the pair of lovers, tend to their nest. The road is lined with herbaceous vegetation that is populated with bees, butterflies, and all manner of winged and crawling folk.

As part of my working vacation, I had the honour and pleasure to be guest speaker at the January 7th, Southwest Florida Ostomy Support Group in Fort Myers, Florida, USA, and with the January 14th, Port Charlotte Ostomy Support Group. It was great fun meeting so many ostomates/caregivers, partaking in the fellowship of the bag. Thank you Howard, Gloria, and the many ostomates who graciously opened their meetings and hearts to me, Percy and Mark. It was a pleasure meeting everyone.

In addition, January brought a message from "Tidings Magazine", (Colostomy Association – UK), I am featured as the Winter 2014, issue 32 cover story, "Pathways to a Colostomy" column, (page 12). I even made the cover. Yes, that's me and Percy walking up the path, and a close up head shot of me. I read each publication of Tidings Magazine as they are published. Tidings provides a platform for sharing interesting and important information that is valuable for all ostomates, caregivers, and medical professionals. Go to www.colostomyassociation.org.uk for information and Tidings Magazine reading pleasure.

But, alas as life will have it, not all is well in paradise. While sitting by the pool Thursday, writing the latest instalment of the sequel to; "Better With A Bag Than In A Bag", (due to be published later this year), 3:00 p.m. arrived and I began to feel unwell, my right ear had started to hurt.

By 9:00 p.m. that evening I was in agony. The right side of my head, my ear, my face, jaw and throat throbbed. As the night progressed the pain intensified. I did not know if I was in the midst of a medical or a dental issue.

At 3:00 a.m. I determined it was a dental emergency. With a one sided chipmunk profile emerging, I felt that if my head exploded it would be a welcome relief. We called our travel medical insurance, and went on the internet to locate the closest emergency dental office. We found one within a 5 minute drive from our location. Thank you for small mercies.

On the Friday morning we parked the car in the parking lot and waited till the door was unlocked at 8:00 a.m. The folks inside were so very personable and professional. Within about 40 minutes I was x-rayed and then examined.

The dentist felt the tooth was finished and dental surgery/ tooth extraction was required. Unfortunately, the infection level was such that she decided we could not proceed until I had some anti-biotic medication in my system. With a compassionate demeanour, she apologized to me, and then wrote out the prescriptions for the much needed antibiotics and pain killers, and scheduled the work to be done on the following day, (Saturday), at 12:30 p.m.

Filling the prescription and starting them immediately, by mid-afternoon the agony in my head turned to misery. Misery being more bearable. My one sided chipmunk profile increased and turned an interesting shade of red. 12:30 p.m. could not come fast enough. It was a long and miserable night.

Arriving for my appointment, I was more than ready for the blessed relief that the extraction of #30 molar, 2nd from the jaw hinge, on the bottom right side would bring.

My compassionate dentist and her assistant attended to me, and began the procedure. The molar was stubborn requiring that it be broken in two and then extracted in 2 pieces. The good news; there were no wayward tooth fragments to remove, it was a clean extraction, and now I am free of the offending tooth.

Given a further anti-biotic and pain killing prescriptions it was back to the condo to recover. The whole evening I remained in misery, hurting from the top of my head to just below my shoulder blades.

I'm on a soft food diet for the next 48 hours, whoopee. And, I finally had a good sleep. Today I have now progressed from misery to plain "yuk". Everything is relative, yuk is so much better than agony and misery. Percy Stoma, the little pooper trooper is bracing for one of the potential side effects of the anti-biotic, diarrhea. Hang in there Percy!

I am awaiting the tooth fairy with great anticipation, and my chipmunk profile is now not so prominent.

Well, interesting beginning of a new year. With much anticipation and fanfare we ring it in. We make plans, and then life gets in the way. That's life. I guess the bottom line is; the sun always shines, but sometimes it's on the other side of the clouds.

Jo-Ann L. Tremblay
Ostomate
"Everyone you meet has a story to tell."

Happy Birthday & Goodbye – *March 11, 2014*

We've just arrived home from 2 months in Florida, while there our family and friends endured the chill of a dark winter, as we basked in the warmth of bright warm days.

During our stay down south my son celebrated his birthday and his son celebrated his birthday, as well. Happy birthday to our beautiful boys.

As life would have it, my dear Auntie passed away. She is much loved by me, goodbye dear lady.

Warm and cold, life and death. Some looking forward and some looking back. The theme for me seems to be duality this past month. This has brought me to the place of deep thinking and deep feeling, yet again. People such as myself who are survivors and have been given another chance at life often experience a great depth of realization. Our near death experience at the apex of one speck in time gives us the opportunity from that day forward to see life and death for what they are in all their mysteries and intricate interrelations. We now have a vantage point from which we can look over the landscape of our existence to see the line between life and death is defined and marked.

So, the theme is duality and what does this mean in our daily lives and in the grand scheme of things? I do think the best place to start is by understanding what duality means. According to one of the online dictionary meanings I came across in my research states; "an instance of opposition or contrast between two concepts or two aspects of something; a dualism".

As an artist and a photographer I often capitalize on the dualities of light and dark, on stillness and movement. In life during this past month I have been exposed to the duality of cold and warm, life and death. During this time I have engaged in the celebrations of life for both of the living in my life, and the one who has passed. I am once again learning that as a mere human I want to keep the one that is called living, and reject the other that is referred to as passing. Yet, the truth is we cannot have one without the other, there is no life without death, and there is death without life. The point that brings it altogether is celebration.

The celebration is the struggle, pleasure and rejoicing of life and the life lived. And so, as a survivor among a multitude of survivors in this world, no matter our circumstances, life can be celebrated. The individualized magic of life lies in our determination to go beyond survival to thrive, to express who we are through our thoughts, words, and actions.

Percy is a stoma and I've had to adjust to him both physically and psychologically. Percy is a symbolic representative of terrible and lousy life happenings for anyone. Everyone has their own individualized version of suffering and loss. Yet we celebrate, because as a stoma Percy is my ticket to life, without him I no longer exist. Without Percy I would not have witnessed and enjoyed the weddings of children, the birth of grandchildren, the love of my life partner, and..., and..., and..., and many other examples of the dualities of life.

Life can be so confusing and downright difficult with the up and down, in and out, success and failure, and the dualities that is the living experience of the nature of the universe and our lives. So far in my life experience learning, by the very fact I'm alive, I will be consistently handed dual experiences. Some will be good and some will be bad. The key to my version of surviving and stepping beyond to thrive through and beyond them is to know a duality when I see it, and to make the time I have, a celebration of life!

Jo-Ann L. Tremblay
Ostomate
"Everyone you meet has a story to tell."

It's Not Taboo, It's Only Poo – *April 2, 2014*

Jo-Ann and I, didn't come up with this blog title it's actually a saying a fellow ostomate shared with members of the Colostomy Association Facebook Group, in celebration of "Bowel Cancer Awareness". I'm a stoma and Jo-Ann is my ostomate, we're one of millions worldwide and many of us are feeling stigmatized, and many ostomates themselves seem to impose stigma upon themselves.

So, when did poo become taboo? What does stigma have to do with a life saving and life sustaining creation? As a stoma I'm simply a "now" end portion of Jo-Ann's colon, and I'm situated to and through the abdominal wall. Imagine for a moment, that the normal exit of poo from the body came from the lower front torso, where I'm located. Under these conditions, disease necessitated surgery that caused the normal frontal exit to be moved to the location of the anus, would this produce a corresponding disgust response?

Well, apparently hearing from numerous folks and speaking with other stomas and their ostomates, the answer is most probably, yes.

This is compelling to Jo-Ann and I, because we live just as heartily as anyone else. There is no shame in what happened. We are bigger than our poo, and how it is eliminated. Yet, stigma is part of the experience for many. Stigma is a Greek word, it's origins referred to a type of marking or tattoo that was cut or burned into the skin of criminals, slaves, or traitors in order to visibly identify them as blemished or morally polluted person. These individuals were to be avoided or shunned, particularly in public places.

Oh my, social stigmas are not only experienced by ostomates, it can occur in many different forms such as; culture, obesity, gender, race, disease, to name a few. And, many people who have been stigmatized feel as though they are transforming from a whole person to a tainted one. The stigmatized whether imposed by others or by themselves, become oppressed and alienated. This can prevent some from seeking help/support, denying themselves access to support networks.

We were recently contacted by a family member of a newly created ostomate. The family member was very concerned as their ostomate was so devastated and embarrassed about their ostomy situation, the potentially vibrant person they could be during and after recovery is now a self imposed "shut-in". The individual will not leave the house, they do not want anyone to visit them, and their self-esteem/self-concept is extremely low. They are recovering from a serious illness that necessitated the creation of the ostomy, and now must adapt and adjust to the ostomy. The family is very concerned about their well-being, and are searching for ways on how they can support their ostomate out of self-stigmatization. People who experience stigma including self-stigmatization experience it as a barrier that can affect nearly every aspect of life, limiting their opportunities, including self-image/self-concept.

Social stigma can occur in stealthy ways, as we found out when we recently exhibited a portrait of me, with our arts group. Jo-Ann is a water colour artist and decided to try her hand at oil painting during her recovery from the surgery that created me. She had pondered what her first painting would be, and it dawned on her; since I had inspired her – and they say when an individual starts any new venture, one should start with what they know – she decided on "Percy, A Self Portrait". Yes, she painted me. The portrait eventually became the cover art for her book, *"Better With a Bag Than In a Bag"*. Now, stoma's are often referred to as rosebuds, this comes about due to the fact that stoma's look somewhat like a rosebud. Nothing ugly or disgusting about a rosebud, or one would think. Well, with much enthusiasm on the, "Share your art" evening, Jo-Ann proudly placed her portrait of me on the pedestal, she looked out to the crowded room to discuss the portrait and back story. Well, the moment they were told it was me , her stoma, ostomy equipment and abdomen as the subject of the painting it was amazing to see the expression on the faces of many of her fellow artists. Jo-Ann noticed eyebrows lowered, noses wrinkled, and many lips became pressed together. Oh goodness, not all, but many of the audience members had a look of disgust on their faces. Jo-Ann quickly informed them that a stoma is often referred to as a rosebud. She then turned the picture upside down and voila the audience saw a beautiful rosebud instead of a stoma. Same picture, different orientation. Jo-Ann noticed a change of facial expressions that were instant, some were of pleasure, some with a look of relief, others of admiration, and there was a sprinkle of nervous laughs. In the question and answer segment, a fellow artist asked Jo-Ann why she had painted the rosebud in a downward facing position. Jo-Ann explained that she had painted the stoma in the orientation that it actually is, you see I point down towards her toes. The artist recommended to Jo-Ann she should keep the picture flipped to the upside down position so that the image looked like the nice rosebud.

The perceived image of the rosebud was acceptable even pleasant to the folks, and the same image displayed as a stoma evoked discomfort for many and even disgust by some. As a painted image I did not receive equitable treatment.

The subject of stigma is powerful, and needs to be understood. Human dignity is the idea that all humans have an inherent worth to be treated with respect regardless of disease, race, gender, nationality, culture, body alterations or any other divisions.

There is so much more exploration we would like to engage in on the issue of stigma. *"Break down the barriers and together we will open the way to dignity for all lives."*

Percy Stoma
Eol. Poopology (**E**xperience **of L**ife)
"Better with a bag than in a bag"

2 Guys, A Canoe & The Big X – *April 23, 2014*

The splash of the paddle on the mirror-calm water triggers a haunting cry of a loon which echoes across the lake as the canoe gently glides through the water. Looking to the land, the tall pines wave in the wind, the water ripples slightly and the sun dapples the soft forest floor in a myriad of colours. Caught up in the rugged beauty and anticipating the crackling of the evenings bonfire, the sinking sun sets just in time to open up the nighttime sky heavy with twinkling stars, together reflecting with the silver magic of the moon across the black water. This is the mystery, awe, and fascination of.... Oh yes, excuse Percy and I as we shake our head awake and re-member, 2 guys, a canoe, and the big X.

Well, it all started a few months ago, Percy and I were thrilled to receive the invitation to be one of the guest speakers at the annual, "Ostomy Toronto Authors Night". We eagerly antici-pated our special evening because it meant we would have another opportunity for ostomy sharing, awareness, advocacy and most of all, to meet new friends. We certainly were not disappointed. Everyone was so inviting and helped us and my husband Mark, feel part of the ostomy community of Toronto. Thank you Ostomy Toronto.

During the meeting we were pleased to be introduced to Ja-son Boyd, who enthusiastically discussed how he and fellow ostomate Jim Fitzgerald have signed up for the Muskoka X challenge, to raise money for children who have ostomies or other special related needs (intermittent catheterization; uri-nary or bowel incontinence due to birth defects, trauma or disease); internal pouch, Crohns disease, Cecostomy Tube or Ulcerative Colitis, Spinal Bifida), to attend the United Ostomy Association of Canada (UOAC) Youth Camp. These young folks are able to participate in summer camp activities with the full freedom and understanding of their camp mates, and professional supervision. A bright and welcoming place for a young person to be confident there is the right kind of support, as they are surrounded by other young folk who can relate.

Oh wow, I remember spending many summers enjoying summer camp. Oh, the swimming, camping out, canoeing, arts and crafts, dancing, youthful hijinks, and the loads of friends I made through the years. What an amazing opportunity for these young folk. Mark, Percy and I have caught the enthusiasm bug.

Firstly, the camp: The United Ostomy Association of Canada, (UOAC) Youth Camp is set up for young people aged 9-18. In addition to wonderful summer camp activities, anatomy and physiology, self-esteem and coping, is also offered. The camp encourages independence and self-confidence with personal care as they enjoy camp activities. The camp also provides individual Enterostomal Therapists, and UOAC counselling on physical and psychosocial needs. Camp Horizon, is located at Bragg Creek, Alberta, Canada, (southwest of Calgary). For more information contact the UOAC office at info1@ostomy-canada.ca.

Now for 2 guys, a canoe & the big X: Huntsville, Ontario, Canada, September 12-14, Jason Boyd and Jim Fitzgerald, both with a permanent ileostomy, will paddle four lakes and two river systems of the Muskoka region. They will face up to 19 portages, and will navigate using only topographic maps, compass, and grid coordinates. They will carry all of their equipment, ostomy equipment, nutrition, and hydration required for the entire race. They will be completely self-sufficient, with no outside assistance, support teams, and no re-supplies. They will paddle 130 km in under 24 hours, on this longest single-day paddling event of its kind in the world. Oh, by the way, "X" is for Expedition.

Jason and Jim, have taken on the Muskoka X in an effort to raise funds to send kids with ostomies and like needs to the UOAC Youth Camp. They are taking on this challenge to help youths get the best life experiences that a camp can give them. Through the sale of limited edition camouflage sponsorship bracelets, you can join Jason and Jim as they take on the Muskoka X race to raise the funds, with a $25,000 goal, on June 21, 2014, Jason and Jim will begin with a 40 km canoe race, and then, September 12-14, a 24 hour 130 km canoe race. For more information, view their Facebook page at: GI J's No Guts, No Glory 2 guys 2 ostomies 130 km race, or go to ostomycanada.akarisin.com/nogutsnoglory.

Nibbling on some blue berries, looking down the white water of the remote waterfall, standing atop the grey stone plateau, a Pike lazily swimming in the glistening water below, the sounds of a crow cawing in the distance……..

Jo-Ann L. Tremblay
Ostomate
"Everyone you meet has a story to tell."

Adventures of the Shocked – *May 21, 2014*

During the first few weeks after I was created, Jo-Ann was mortified at just about everything about me. I remember her lying in bed with a drain tube in her abdomen, intravenous lines in her veins, and me, all red, swollen and raw. "Oh my God, what's happened to me, I'm scared", rampaged through her mind. When my bag and flange were removed to change to fresher equipment, "I poop in a bag!", were the next set of words that screamed inside of her.

Here I am as ugly as I am, yet, I'm the very thing that keeps her alive, and I have to wear a bag over me, not by choice but by necessity. What a shock all of this was to her, part of what had always been inside her body, was now on the outside, (I'm her outdoor plumbing, so to speak), she now has to live the rest of her life with the daily discomforts and concerns of an ostomate, whilst dealing with the occasional output breaches that can happen at any time during the day and night, just to mention a few of her challenges.

So many changes occur for anyone and everyone when they must face illness, a significant emotional event, or life alterations, chosen or thrust upon them, ostomates are no exception. Often feeling trapped by life conditions, people experience a form of the grieving process. Research tells us the process goes like this; 1. Shock and denial, 2. Pain and guilt, 3. Anger and bargaining, 4. Depression, reflection and loneliness, 5. The upward turn, 6. Reconstruction and working through, 7. Acceptance and hope. The key to success is to know and believe grief is not a place, that it is actually a process. Time does not heal, but, it takes time to heal the body, mind, emotions and the human spirit.

With this in mind Jo-Ann and I set out to create and embrace our new normal, whatever the heck that was going to be. Jo-Ann gave herself permission, and fully surrendered to the grieving process. She immersed herself in the pain and guilt, she wallowed in her loneliness, was a full participant in her pity parties held daily at a particular point in time. She couldn't go back, she couldn't change anything. No one could fix her nor her situation, no one could do anything in particular, what she really needed was to know she is cared for and support-ed.

She was once again launched in a giant world, where the people she knew at the time didn't understand anything she was living through, they didn't know the half of it. She spent copious amounts of energy trying to keep things going and contained. Eventually she began to feel for all the amazing people out there navigating life altering challenges no matter what they are, and realized she was not alone. Eventually she began to change the way she saw her and everyone's life. She embraced the perception that people can shape the way they create and experience life, come what may. A profound change in perspective allows people to see themselves and their lives with clarity, and this fuels their courage to alter their thoughts and approach to experiencing it. They have the power to change their perception of themselves and their lives, in spite of it all.

The truth and authenticity of whatever it is that has struck in a person's life, like a bolt of lightning cannot be erased. In our case, Jo-Ann is still an ostomate. I am for the rest of her life

outside her body, she will continue to live with the daily discomfort and concerns of an ostomate, whilst dealing with the
occasional output breaches at any time during the day and
night, just to mention a few of her challenges. It's tedious and
filled with the occasional resentment, and the moments of
transformative triumph.

This is not a place were we stand stuck, it's a process, and
I'm a part of this remarkable journey. Together with my stoma
life-sustaining abilities, (a superhero in my own estimation),
and Jo-Ann's commitment to live a joyous and full life, in spite
of it all, together we weave a tapestry we conceive as a
whole, working together as a team. This is the way it is for us,
we cannot go back, we cannot change the past, we cannot
take away the disease that started all of this, what we can do
is put one foot in front of the other and continue on our way.

Percy Stoma
Eol. Poopology (**E**xperience **o**f **L**ife)
"Everyone you meet has a story to tell."

Top Of The Chart Hits – *June 17, 2014*

The spring of 2014 has been a kaleidoscope of emotions. In the past 8 weeks, we buried 3 family members, and, a dear friend of ours. Dark clouds raced throughout our emotions. Then, the sun came out and we welcomed the birth of our 5th grandchild. We have taken the sunshine with the clouds. Oh, life can be so adventurous.

Every day all of us who are left, have the opportunity to take hold of ourselves and lives, to embrace the good and not so good, come what may. Each day is a beginning again. For those of us who are ostomates, the creation of our ostomies marked the defining moment of our 2nd chance at life, our beginning again. As we take care of our individual ostomy, at any given time of the day or night on a daily basis, we are continuously reminded of the reality and magnificence of beginnings again and of, keeping on.

I am alive, and when I survived my life saving surgery that created my buddy, "Percy", I fought hard to be part of this world. I had high ambitions. I was not going to miss a moment, an event, circumstance, nor happening, no matter the depth or the height of the life experience. Life is a mix of ups and downs, and each brings to our lives all the colour and textures conscious living can bring. Our individual worlds are all the more interesting and sometimes with a lot of work, will eventually be better for it. Even in the most challenging of times, there are nuggets of gold that brings delight to us, when we open our hearts and minds.

My "Top of the Chart Hits" for the past 8 weeks are:

Although we buried one Aunt and two Uncles, I had the distinct honour of being with my beloved cousins and family members. We laughed and cried together. Due to living in scattered parts of the country, it isn't often we can all get together and have the opportunity to rekindle and reconnect our relationships.

Our delighted 5-year-old grandson told us his breakfast menu, but his very favourite was, "peanut butter with toast on it."

Our maturing 12-year-old grandson called and said, "I love you Gramma Jo. I miss you, I'd like to come over and hang out with you and Dramps." My response, "we miss you to honey, we're going over to your place for dinner in about 2 hours, we'll see you then." "But Gramma Jo, I really want to hang out with just you and Dramps", he pleaded. "Well, of course honey, we'll pick you up in about 10 minutes", I promised. We did pick him up, he brought his favourite game, he then taught it his Dramps and I, and we had a delightful 2 hours just hanging out.

"Hey, do you want to take a walk with me Gramma Jo?", asked our 9-year-old granddaughter. "Sure honey", said I. "I know where north, south, east and west is Gramma Jo", she said at about 5 minutes into our walk. "That's terrific honey, even though you may not know where you are in any given moment, you'll always know where you came from, and the direction you want to go. Good for you", I said as I admired her clever mind.

Happy Father's Day, Dad!

What a beautiful picture of our son, (daddy), and 3-year-old granddaughter (now big sister), cuddled together embracing and welcoming their newborn, our baby granddaughter.

My husband able to hang up his cane and walk without pain following a severe bout with gout.

Planning an adventure for my sister's 60th birthday celebration of life.

Well, these are the top of the chart hits in my life over the past 8 weeks. As I woke up to another beginning again day, we received a text from our youngest daughter who resides in another country, it read, "my baby bump is showing!". Every life is tough, but, every life has its top of the chart hits. The adventure continues.....

Jo-Ann L. Tremblay
Ostomate
"Everyone you meet has a story to tell."

Walk A Mile In Other Shoes – *July 15, 2014*

A while ago my husband and I were taking a short vacation to visit our newborn granddaughter. We stopped at a roadside rest stop that offered various food chains for refreshments, and restroom facilities for travellers. In my excitement to meet our new little one, Percy became rather active, as sometimes happens to all of us when we experience positive or negative stress.

I headed for the restroom, as I knew I would have to change some of my ostomy equipment. I eyed the "wheelchair accessible" cubical which would provide Percy and I with a little extra room and sink facilities within the cubical, which we could really use for organizing, removing and handling our used flange/bag, and for applying the fresh new equipment efficiently and discreetly.

When finished I exited the cubical, and it was at this point a lady began to speak to me harshly and very loudly. Loudly, I assumed so that everyone in the restroom would notice me. She stated, "Those cubicles are for people who are handicapped. They need them and you're wasting the space. I would think better and more respectful in the future, if I were you!" Caught by surprise, my first thought was, who appointed you the bathroom cubicle police?

After a couple of deep breaths I settled in and allowed her the opportunity to vent at me and finish her aggressive desire to put me in my place, according to her private logic. Meanwhile, I stood straight and tall, (well as tall as a 4 foot 11 inch woman can stand), and maintained eye contact with her.

A part of me congratulated her in my mind and heart. Here she was championing for any potential person who may require the wheelchair accessible cubical, that she felt that I without reason and certainly with disrespect had used and could have caused distress for another. My next thought was, I'm sure most folks in a wheelchair can speak for themselves. Then, the other part of my mind felt frustrated with her ignorance of what the situation Percy and I were in, and her need to publicly humiliate us.

When she was finished my only response in a quiet voice that I directed to her was; "There are some challenges that are not as visible as others are." Then, I lifted my shirt a bit and lowered the waistband of my shorts just a little, enough so that she could see the very top of Percy's ostomy equipment. I then simply walked out of the restroom facility holding my head high.

In one way I could see where she was coming from. What she failed to remember in the restroom that day was, "Don't judge a person until you have walked a mile in their shoes." The earliest source of this enlightening wisdom I can find dates to the Cherokee people. Nelle Harper Lee, an American author was seemingly inspired by the saying in her book, "To Kill a Mockingbird", where she wrote:

"You never really know a man until you understand things from his point of view, until you climb into his skin and walk around in it."

The graphic restroom incident is a grand life lesson, a reminder for Percy, myself and for all people, to be mindful that before we criticize another we should take the time to think ourselves into another person's shoes, as we endeavour to be compassionate and empathetic.

Being able to empathize is the ability to identify and understand another person's feelings without experiencing them for yourself at that particular moment. The ability to literally experience the world from another person's perspective, to walk in their shoes, to view life from their living conditions and to feel what it feels like to be that person.

As I mentioned, part of my mind and heart felt encouraged that any visibly physically challenged person who may have entered the restroom would be championed by someone. In that moment I tried to see her from her vantage point, from where she viewed me exiting the cubicle with no visible physical challenge. I worked hard to leave my opinion of her aggressive behaviour aside for that short moment, no matter how arrogant and full of herself she appeared to me on the surface. While in this state of unbiasedness I was able to assume she thought herself as a champion, and that was probably behind her behaviour. I gave her a brief and partial glimpse of my ostomy equipment that also exposed a small part of my extensive abdominal scarring from multiple major surgeries, as I felt it was only fair for her to share in the grand lesson with us, that she had precipitated. I have always felt that everyone has a story to tell, and I would like to add for today, "take the time to walk in their shoes, even for just a moment."

Jo-Ann L. Tremblay
Ostomate
"Everyone you meet has a story to tell, take the time to walk in their shoes, even for just a moment."

Percy and I are pleased to announce, the United Ostomy Association of Canada, (UOAC), has a new redesigned website, you can view it at ostomycanada.ca. The UOAC welcomes everyone to grab a cup of coffee or tea, relax and spend some time with them as you explore their website.

A Celebration Of Life – *July 21, 2014*

Today is a day of celebration for Percy Stoma and I. It was 3 years ago today I was at the brink of death as I underwent lifesaving surgery, and little Percy was created.

It's our celebration of life day. A 2nd chance at life is the icing on the cake, the cherry on top!

Have a most excellent day everyone, enjoy each moment of it, and celebrate who you are.

"Jo-Ann"

"Yes Percy"

"We're going to party all day till I get pooped out, aren't we?"

"Yap Percy, we sure are."

Happy day everyone!

Jo-Ann L. Tremblay & Percy Stoma
"Everyone you meet has a story to tell."

Vive la différence – *August 11, 2014*

The newest news about ostomates I've noticed, is the trend in breaking the taboo of ostomies and ostomy bags through posted photographic images.

Facebook, Instagram and Twitter are just a few of the social media being used by ostomates to show and share their colostomy, ileostomy, urostomy bags and scars.They are young, middle-aged, elderly, male, female, and all of them are plucking up the courage to share themselves and their bags to wider and wider audiences.

I have heard some folks, (ostomates and non-ostomates) take offence to the photographic images, and I heard other folks cheering them on. Aspiring model ostomate Bethany Townsend posted her image with Crohns and Colitis UK Facebook group with her story, and the photos went viral. (See more at http://tiny.cc/6rofkx).

Then there's male model Blake Beckford (33) from Stratford-upon-Avon, who suffered from ulcerative colitis, eventually his colon was removed and he has a permanent ileostomy. He had dreamed of becoming a fitness model before his 2003 diagnosis and after 10 years, he developed the confidence to pursue his ambitions, and he has landed a feature in Men's Health Magazine. (See more at http://tiny.cc/bwfkx)

These brave ostomates are working to make news as a way of getting ostomy attention, support, and for spreading awareness. The tracks laid by ostomates everywhere is one of a trend that other industries are now climbing aboard and riding the vive la différence train. JC Penny for example is featuring disabled models in a recent campaign. The major retailer states they are committed to greater representation in the fashion industry, representing their diverse range of customers. To date I don't believe they are featuring an ostomate, but who knows what next year will bring.

Then there's Jessica Grossman, (24), of Ontario, Canada, who is a trailblazing campaigner for women with ostomies, inspiring them to embrace their 'second chance at life' through her initiatives. (See more at: Facebook – Uncover Ostomy).

Photo-based activities conducted by oneself or as part of an organized group or project is occurring in many forms of community settings, and are catalysts for political/social change and for community-strengthening. Ostomates sharing their images and stories is an important step in allowing people to take pride in and ownership of their ostomy, building confidence and supporting their feelings of validation that they are being listened to and taken seriously.

In my understanding, the images I have seen represent a means to an end rather than an end itself, for the purpose of emphasizing their courage and well being rather than illness. They are sharing to engage in awareness, advocacy and possibly their own individual healing. The images provide opportunities for peer support, socializing with new people, (ostomates and non-ostomates), and personal support. Sharing the ostomates realities is a way we can all be more understanding of one another, regardless of any differences we my have.

Percy and I feel this new and inspiring trend is an opportunity to send out a resounding cheer, "go ahead folks, be proud of who you are, you're amazing, embrace your ostomy, inspire others, and keep spreading the awareness.

Matters Of The Heart & The Case Of The Missing Teddy – *September 29, 2014*

Here I am snuggled up to her, my dear ostomate, I'm all warm and safely tucked in. The family room air conditioning is blowing cool air down on us, on an already cool day. Breakfast finished, her 80 year old Mother is reading the morning paper. With every turn of a page, the sound of crinkling newspaper brings back memories of her childhood. Then, her mother's hair was light brown, now her silvery white hair glistens in the golden glow of the lamplight.

Her sister is reading a book that must be at least 1000 pages thick. It has a beige cover with a dark brown spine. One of her old and much loved literary treasures. With each word she reads about angels and healing, she reminds Jo-Ann of a cat in a pool of sunshine curled up in the bulky chair. Every once in a while she closes her eyes and takes a short nap.

Her husband Mark, sits in the tapestry covered chair, the musician and high tech wizard is reading another biography on his ebook reader.

The TV from the other room is filling the air with the muffled chitter chatter of the morning news program. The last super moon till 2015 is now fully set, and a sunrise is spreading it's rays into an azure sky. All of this brings sweetness to the beginning a new day. Yet, we are a family in fear. We are family with optimism. We are a family together without one.

I'm Percy Stoma, and me and my family are sitting in the "family room" of the Heart Institute in Ottawa, Canada. The University of Ottawa Heart Institute, (UOHI), is Canada's

largest cardiovascular health centre. A complete cardiac centre, encompassing prevention, diagnosis, treatment, rehabilitation, research, and education. The UOHI was founded by
Dr. Wilbert J. Keon. The Order of Canada recipient, was the
first Canadian to implant an artificial heart into a human as a
bridge to transplant. It is the Institute that is world renowned
for many other procedural and technical heart saving and life
enhancing break throughs.

From the volunteers who greeted us at the main entrance, the
medical professionals, (nurses, technicians, and doctors), and
even the custodial staff, with their beating hearts expressed
all of the heart felt care, concern, competency and profes-
sionalism a family needs at a time like this, a time when our
loved ones life hangs in the balance.

You see, Jo-Ann's Dad is at this moment undergoing open
heart surgery. Our patriarch is 80 years young, a man who
has always kept himself in top physical condition. We are in
shock as he's the last person we would have thought would
be in the operating theatre, undergoing triple bypass surgery.

He's a force of nature, a man who has been our mentor. And,
in this moment the landscape is dramatically different. We are
adrift. We are in the middle of nowhere, and at the same time
somewhere we never expected to be.

It's Jo-Ann's second chance at life, I her Percy Stoma is the
biological mechanism she relies on to stay alive and present
right now with her beloved family. The people she most wants
to be with, in a place and a circumstance she doesn't want to
be at. Life – hmm… throws curves, zingers, and how many
left turns does a person take in a lifetime. Sure would be nice
if a person is born with all the coping tools to get through it all

like a breeze. Well, as George Gershwin (famous musician and composer) put it, "Life is a lot like jazz – it's best when you improvise".

So here we are, improvising, as the hours are ticking by. With the family snuggled in the "family room", on the surface it's almost a sweet and dreamy scene. Then, the cardiac surgeon fills the doorway of the room, and like a blaring alarm his presence shakes us awake. "The surgery went well. Quicker than we planned. He's now in the Intensive Care Unit, (ICU). It will be a few hours more, and then you'll be able to visit him", he said.

SWEET!

DELICIOUS!

During the following days we switched to a recovery mode that carried us day by day to the happy place. But, as Jo-Ann's life experience has never been conventional, another one of life's curves lay just ahead, lying in wait for her.

Her Dad was now on the 3rd floor of the Heart Institute. Amazing Earth Angels in the guise of nurses mostly, and Doctor's, had been attending to our beloved for 5 days post surgery, now. It was early Saturday morning when Mark awakened with pain and heaviness in his chest. With a shot of nitroglycerin (nitro), which opens up (dilates) the arteries in the heart, (coronary arteries), under his tongue, he waited five minutes. The discomfort abated for a short time, and then it returned. He administered a second shot of nitro. The pain and heaviness subsided. He suggested he should stay home and relax.

Jo-Ann said, "no-no-no, you're not going to be alone when you're feeling like this. We're picking up Mom and Diane, and heading to the Institute to be together with Dad. You're not going to be alone, and besides which, the Heart Institute is the best place to be if you have another episode."

So off we went. Well, as life would have it, on route Mark began to experience another episode. Keeping all of this quiet in order to spare our family from additional stress at this time. We arrived at hospital and into the room we quickly entered. Jo-Ann devised a bit of a ruse and explained to her Dad, that she had not been able to take her usual morning walks, and I needed these walks to help keep me flowing, and so, she was going to take a walk, and Mark was coming with her.

Jo-Ann, Mark and I walked out to the nurses station, and Mark said to one of the staff, "You're not going to believe this, but, I've had to administer two separate shots of nitro this morning, and I'm not feeling very well."

They promptly sat him in a wheelchair and rushed him across the hospital campus to the Emergency Department of the Civic Hospital. During the following hours, Mark was now hooked up to monitors which were keeping a close watch on his vitals, and he required two more shots of nitro to fully stabilize him.

He was admitted to the Heart Institute, and now tucked into his bed in a ward on the 5th floor. We are a family in fear. We are an optimistic family. We are a family together without two.

In the days that followed, JoAnn, myself and family rode the elevators between the 3rd and 5th floors. Jo-Ann's Dad was concerned for his son-in-law. He could fully relate to Mark's situation and feeling he wanted to reach out, had a vase of flowers with a little white teddy bear delivered upstairs from him to Mark.

A grateful, delighted and touched Mark, took pictures of the flowers and teddy, so that Jo-Ann's Dad would be able to see them.

A couple of days later, Jo-Ann's Dad was discharged home to the care of her mother and sister, while Jo-Ann and I continued our daily trek to the Institute for our Mark. Many tests were conducted, all was quiet for Mark, and there were no other episodes.

UNTIL!

Jo-Ann and I had been sleeping at night with the phone on the pillow beside her head, when all of a sudden we were awakened at 4:00 am, by the ringing of the phone. The nurse on the other end of the line stated, "Mark has had an eventful night, and is now being moved to the 1st floor, into the Coronary Care Unit. He is stable and if there is any other concerns, we'll call you immediately.

In our state of emotion, I became a little overactive, hmm... sorry Jo-Ann, I just couldn't hold back.

We arrived at the Coronary Care Unit on the 1st floor, after getting into the elevator and pressing the button for the 5th floor. Then, realizing she had pressed the wrong button, Jo-Ann promptly pressed the 3rd floor button, only to realize as the elevator doors opened, that she really wanted to press the 1st floor button. Geez!

Arriving into a room that looked just short of the ICU, we saw a rosy-faced and smiling Mark. After his cheery and affectionate greeting, he stated, "I don't know where my teddy is. He didn't arrive with me."

When Mark had started the episode at about 3:30 am earlier that morning, there had been a flurry of activity as the monitoring instruments were sounding off. There were alarms that could be heard throughout the 5th floor. Nurses and Doctors had jumped into controlled and coordinated action. Mark's lovely ward mates in the other beds were very concerned and worried for Mark, who was in the process of being stabilized and then hustled from the ward room to the 1st floor.

The nurses had gathered all of Mark's clothing and what not, during the excitement to be moved with him. But as it was, the flowers and teddy had not moved with him. Teddy was missing in action. He had disappeared, he was no where to be seen.

When I was satisfied I could leave Mark for a short while, I headed up to the 5th floor to relay to Mark's ward compatriots that he was fine, and to locate his missing teddy. The fella's were relieved to hear about Mark, but no one had seen teddy.

We excused ourselves and went back to the first floor, pressing the correct elevator button this time. Later that day we popped back up to the 5th floor to check in on the fella's and to give them Mark's health report. It was at this time a concerned nurse apologized to me, she could not find teddy anywhere.

Mark's former ward mates, with sadness in their voices, told us they and the nurses had looked for teddy, and the little fella was no where to be found. You see, Mark had told them who the flowers and teddy had come from, about his father-in-law, and so, they knew how important teddy is.

We assured everyone that although we regret the loss of teddy, we are so grateful for the compassion and understanding of what teddy represents to us. And, we are grateful for their "all out 5th floor and elevator search", for the little white fella. With a wave good bye we headed down the hall to the, yes, elevators, yet another time.

As we passed the nurses station, Jo-Ann turned her head to view all of the many trinkets, gifts and flowers passed on to them by patients and their families. Amongst the myriad of objects, Jo-Ann was surprised to see a little white fuzzy face, whose black eyes twinkled as they reflected the overhead lights, with a half smile peeking out from behind a blue box.

TEDDY!

Snapping him up, sure enough, it was teddy. The nurses broke into broad smiles, Jo-Ann hugged teddy to her chest as she turned around and scampered back down the hall to the ward to show the fella's that teddy has been found. Indeed teddy was intact, and within an elevator ride would once again be safe and sound with Mark.

Later that day Mark underwent an Angiogram that determined that although he's experiencing A-Typical symptoms for a heart issue, his heart and arteries are healthy. The source of the issue lays elsewhere. There are many tests and such ahead of Mark, in order to pinpoint the source.

Today, Dad continues to recover beautifully, Mark is home, and teddy has a special place beside our bed.

In all matters of the heart ; we are forever touched and grateful by the heart felt care expressed to our family by all of the special people at the Heart Institute in Ottawa, Canada. And, speaking heart to heart; this has been an everyday amazing slice of life story. Sure glad I'm here for Jo-Ann doing my stoma duties and attending to my jobbies, so that Jo-Ann can be here for the experiences and times of her life.

Percy Stoma
Eol. Poopology
"Better With a bag than in a bag."

Better WITH A Bag Than In A Bag is now available on KOBO – *October 1, 2014*

We are pleased to announce that not only is "Better With a Bag Than In a Bag"available with Amazon in paperback and on kindle, in Canada, USA, United Kingdom, Australia, Europe and Japan, this compelling tale that speaks to the human spirit, that brought author Jo-Ann L. Tremblay from the brink of death to recovery through humour and inspiration, is now available with KOBO. Check out KOBO at tinyurl.com/ngrlp82. For further information and an additional list of online book dealers offering the book, and how you can purchase your very own copy, just click "Better With a Bag Than In a Bag" at the top of THE OSTOMY FACTOR blog Home Page.

Jo-Ann L. Tremblay
Ostomate
"Everyone you meet has a story to tell."

What We've Lost – What We Have – *October 29, 2014*

So many changes occur for anyone and everyone when they face illness, a significant emotional event, or life alteration(s), whether chosen or thrust upon them. Ostomates such as myself are not an exception, and we at one time had to face all of them.

There are many reasons why a person will undergo surgery to become an ostomate, and none of them are easy. Whatever it was or will happen that will bring a person to a life alteration, they will experience feelings of being bent and broken. Our body, mind, emotions and human spirit screams for a second chance at life.

Whatever our life situation may be, one thing is for sure, none of us can change the past. We cannot take away or erase the incident or circumstance that started everything. What we can do is, put one foot in front of the other, and then continue on our way, in spite of it all.

There are very few of us who are fearless in the face of loss, and the memory of what we once had. With each foot moving forward we march to the beat of our recovery drum, and sway to the rhythm of our new normal, all the while, doing everything possible to shake off the terrible fear.

When a significant emotional event occurs in a lifetime, and every life I know has had at least one, and most often, people have had many, our way of looking at ourselves, our lives, and the people around us is forever changed. Some of us feel trapped by the life altering condition, and for others, we experience a grieving process that eventually leads us to the promise of a full life, even in the face of uncertainty.

All life is fragile and limited. Before our life altering and significant emotional event, (SEE), life wasn't always fair. We didn't know how long our lives would be, no one really knows. We at times lived without peace, and the journey was not always smooth. Then the SEE happened, and we lost somethings, for some of us we even lost the use of body parts. And, we will never look at ourselves and life the same way again. Yet, life is still fragile, limited, and precious. Life isn't always going to be fair. We don't know how long we will live, no really knows. At times we will live without peace, and the journey will not always be smooth.

Before and after our SEE, we navigate along our life path, and it takes a lot of time and work to nourish our body, mind, emotions and human spirit. The potential energy that can fuel our progress lies in discovering the pleasure of living each moment to the fullest. The appreciation of life's smallest pleasures, and the all out, no holds barred grandest of life's happenings. What we've lost is gone.

What we have, is precious and can be easily lost again. Life inhales, and then exhales again. There are times when we feel hurt, isolated, and angry. There are times when we are energized, awake, and alive. We need to allow ourselves to grieve, and even take a time out. And then, SEE a doorway of opportunity opening up, and just walk right through it, come what may.

Jo-Ann L. Tremblay
Ostomate
"Everyone you meet has a story to tell."

Welcome To The Planet – *November 28, 2014*

We are once again awakened from the slumber of life's everyday routine. Through the scramble and the chaos of the language of the body, fuelled by primal energy, our 6th grandchild came out to greet the world this past week.

Our little one who has rocked our world is ready now to be present for a lifetime of lived experience, refracted through the lens of her body, emotion, mind and human spirit experiences.

She enters her story into recorded history. A story that is a unique microcosm of a larger tapestry of family, community, nation and planet. As she grows and develops, she will weave the strands of her individuality into the genetic cloth of her ancestral bloodline with a thread that cannot be broken.

As her grandparent, her presence thoroughly intoxicates me. From the point of view of an ostomate who has captained her ship during a storm of experience, weathered nature's power, and the threat of death, my second chance at life has graced me with you, our sweet little belly fruit.

How exquisite my bonus days have become, I'm now seasoned with sugar, spice and everything nice. I have been given another opportunity to embrace, caress and admire this generation's newest family treasure. Together we will travel upon the wind, as we feel the flutter of fairy wings. We will bounce balls and spin jacks with our sixth sweet and delicious fruit that clings to the family tree.

Welcome to planet Earth, little Liviana. Thank you for joining us at this time. This is my pledge to you and to all of the little ones of your generation, wherever they live in the world who are arriving and those who will come: I as a member of the human family will do all that I can to build a better world for you. I will actively participate in the honouring of every nationality, ethnic group, and gender. Through consistently building upon my own wisdom gained through experience, I will actively contribute to increasing your knowledge as I pass on the learning to you, our next generation. I will assist you in keeping alive the legacy of those who came before you as they are your roots. I will endeavour to provide you with food and other things that are needed to live healthy and that will assist you in growing stronger. In actions and feelings I surround you and hold within, unconditional and pure love, so that you will always know how special and magnificent you truly are.

Thank you for you.

Jo-Ann L. Tremblay
Ostomate
"Everyone you meet has a story to tell."

Food For Thought and The Tastebuds –
December 16, 2014

A recipe for success and gastronomic delights.

The personal and professional issues we deal with in life are universal to everyone, and at the same time, they are experienced uniquely by each person. No matter your struggles, everyone is individually co-creating themselves and their particular life experience. Along with everyone on this planet, you are pursuing goals and meeting challenges in order to achieve health, happiness and prosperity.

In addition to our universal issues, ostomates have their particular challenges to contend with on a daily basis. Our ostomies are a mixed blessing. On one hand they are the medical miracles that give us a second chance at life, promoting wellness, energy, and the opportunity to live life to the fullest, come what may. An ostomy is also a constant reminder of the illness we experienced, and the damage it caused.

Having said this, acceptance of the changes and transition we ostomates experience is fuelled by our attitude. A positive attitude truly helps us transform and settle into our new normal. We know of course this is more easily said than done, but the effort is well worth it, it really does pay off in the long run.

A positive attitude is your success attitude. A success attitude is the drive to empower every act with the intent for fixing anything that is bungling up the hard work you're doing. A person's attitude is a great factor in gaining the confidence of others, and for obtaining desired results. Your attitude will always play an important part in how easy or difficult an experience will be. Your ally throughout your whole life in good times and bad, will be your attitude.

Very often people come up with creative excuses, and these excuses can present major obstacles to success. The best strategy for dealing with excuses is by eliminating them as much as possible. This is a challenge in itself as excuses are seductive. The bonus for eliminating excuses will cause you to be more open to learning from an experience and this will fuel your success attitude.

There really is no simple recipe for success, but there is one essential ingredient and that is - A Success Attitude.

Success Attitude Recipe

Add 1 part *Definite Decision*. Don't just think about it – go for it. A quitter never wins and a winner never quits.

Add 1 part *Commitment*. Go the extra mile. Everything you do, do your best. Your best will bring you closer to your dreams, no matter how menial the task.

Add 1 part *Life Study*. Objectively listen, ask questions, and observe yourself. You will always actively learn from every person you come into contact with, from everything you do, and from every experience.

Mix ingredients together, and place them in a willing mind free from excuses. Feed them to your conscious and subconscious mind till it becomes your individual success attitude.

We are a body, a mind, and we have a human spirit. For a little fun, Percy and I thought we'd like to share a gluten and lactose free recipe to delight your taste buds.

Peanut Butter & Marshmallow Sandwich Cookies

Makes 24 cookies and 12 sandwiches.

Ingredients

1 cup (250 ml) natural peanut butter

1 cup (225 grams) sugar

1 large egg, lightly beaten

1 teaspoon vanilla extract

Marshmallow Fluff (if using)

Instructions

Preheat the oven to F 350 and line baking sheets with parchment paper.

Place all ingredients in a bowl and mix on low until combined. Use a small ice cream or cookie scoop and drop 1 ½ tablespoonful's of dough onto the prepared backing sheets. Use a fork to flatten the mounds of dough and create a criss-cross pattern on each cookie.

Bake cookies for 10-12 minutes or until golden around the edges. Remove from the oven and rest on the baking sheet for a few minutes until the cookies firm up enough to transfer to cooling racks.

Once cooled spread at least 1 heaping tablespoonful of Marshmallow Fluff onto the back on one of the peanut butter cookies and top with another. Enjoy!

In closing as we say goodbye to 2014, Percy Stoma and I extend our best wishes from our home to your home. As you ring in 2015, may the magic of new beginnings fill your home and heart with peace and joy. We sincerely wish that the next year ahead will be your best year yet.

Jo-Ann L. Tremblay
Ostomate
"Everyone you meet has a story to tell."

Year 4

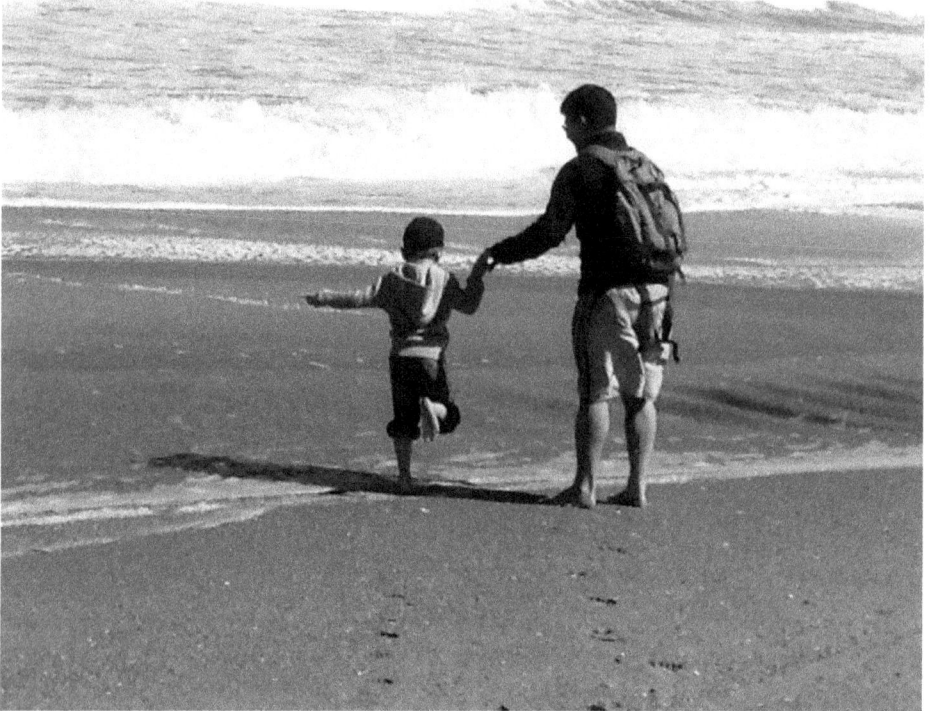

Move on in life and go along with it. Grasp each chance with both hands as they come, and give them the opportunity to come to you.

I have had the distinct pleasure of living and growing up by the ocean for many years of my childhood. My romance with the vast sea nurtured my imagination, emotions, serenity and most of all, educated me in the enigma we call life and living, with all it has to offer. The ocean's eternal motion spawns the tales and legends of life's joys, struggles, and death experiences.

Brave seafaring women and men climb aboard their tiny ships that hold and protect their lives and livelihoods. They set forth on the full tide hoping to glide over shimmering water whose tranquil cadence moves them along. All the while, they scan the distant horizon knowing that at any given time, at any moment indeed, the sea will boil up tumultuous forces filling their ears with grating roars, slapping their faces with wild spray, and the struggle to maintain balance.

Through the security of the bay, up the straight, along the coast and then out to the unknown we navigate. Our journey provokes speculation and fearful anticipation of what may lie ahead. The mystery of the big blue sea is akin to the mystery of our human lives.

2015 was a year where I worked hard at captaining my ship with responsibility and accountability for all aspects of the ship and the journey. I made sure my ship was fit for the journey. I guided the general course of operations and direction that I wanted to take. I prepared for any event, and the protection and well-being of all who were on this journey with me. I worked hard to gain the knowledge, wisdom, and spirit I needed to navigate the year long journey through and throughout the inevitable times of calm and storm.

We are all captains of our ship. Your ship is you, and the ship is on a journey of a lifetime.

And so, ahoy, mateys! This be a fair and true year long set of blog posts to do with life, 13 of them in all. Be fairly warned: I, being an ostomate of the most scurvy sort, will make you chuckle at times, bring a tear to your eye, and will serve up a tankard full of life's brew for your entertainment. So, be there any sea-dogs out there who would like to join in climb aboard, and ye holler from atop the vessels crow's nest and call out, Ahoy!

Of Seagulls, Sand, & Sequels – *January 13, 2015*

"Your whole body, from wingtip to wingtip," Jonathan would say, other times, *"is nothing more than your thought itself, in a form you can see. Break the chains of your thought, and you break the chains of your body, too."* Richard David Bach, (American Writer), Jonathan Livingston Seagull.

We have left the harsh cold of snow-land, the world of white and winter, and have arrived in Florida, eager to listen to the music of the wave-washed coast. We are ready to bask in the warm sunshine, and it is here that I have found the sanctuary that I need to write "the sequel" to, Better With A Bag Than In A Bag.

That narrative is a book I did not originally set out to write. Just a little more than a year before I published it, I had arrived at death's door after a 4 year struggle with illness and suffering. I survived against all odds, it was an amazing triumph of the surgical medical team, home care workers, my caregiver/life partner Mark, my body, and my human spirit. I fully embrace the full and glorious extent of this, and I am in awe.

During that year I was engaged on the battlefields of body recovery. My goal was to transform myself through a spectacular recovery. As I am a writer, one of the ways of clearing my thoughts and laundering my emotions is to write. And so, during that year, on a daily basis, I would write a word, a sentence, or paragraph on how I was feeling, what had happened, what I was experiencing, and where I thought I was.

I felt my light needed to sparkle and shine once again. I had high hopes. I knew I was recovering but didn't know how much recovery would actually occur. Is there a limit; or is it limitless?

Better With A Bag Than In A Bag, chronicles the journey of me, an ordinary person, who had to endure a devastating illness, emergency lifesaving surgery, the creation of Percy, and the year long recovery that brought me to my 1st stom-aversary. On that day, we enjoyed a celebration of life, filled with friends, good eats, and all the sparkle July 21, 2012, could bring.

On the next day, I sat down and read all of the musings, rants, and laughs I had experienced and jotted down in the darkest and lightest of moments during that year. When I had finished reading, I realized that in spite of myself, I had written a book that would become, Better With A Bag Than In A Bag, *From the brink of death to recovery through humour and inspiration*. And, it was also the day that the full impact of reality set in, and I realized that although the official recovery process was now completed, the lingering carnage from the original disease, the damage from the extensive surgery, and the emotional toll it takes to adapt and live with an altered body function, was just beginning.

Percy, my life sustaining stoma and I are at the beginning of our, "beginning again". Hmm…well ah, beginning of what, why, when, where and the how of a new life, new self, a new normal, whatever the heck that's supposed to be, at any rate.

My journey is not complete. No journey I suppose ever is. So, marching to the beat of the recovery drum that sets the pace, I am now writing "the sequel", which will be published later this year. It will be a book in which, together, we will explore the fact that regardless of your life altering occurrence, the truth and authenticity of whatever has struck you like a bolt of lightning cannot be erased. And, one of the key's to success is to know and believe the grief you feel is not a place where you stand stuck. It is a process, a challenging and remarkable journey.

The sequel is about not being bound by physical or social challenges. We all have the ability to get on with life with the cards we have been dealt through strength and determination. Percy is co-writing the book with me. Well, what can I say? That little stoma has an opinion on everything, and we know Percy likes to toot his own horn.

Of seagulls, sand, and sequels in life, we observe from the edge of the waves, a vast ocean of life and possibilities. As Richard Back says in his story – Jonathan Livingston Seagull, *"Break the chains of your thought, and you break the chains of your body, too."*

Jo-Ann L. Tremblay
Ostomate
"Everyone you meet has a story to tell."

Magical First Times – *February 26, 2015*

On a cloudless day a child dances on the warm sand. He sees the ocean, he hears the rhythm of the pounding surf, and he smells the salty air, for the very first time in his life. His daddy takes hold of his hand and they make their way to the edge of the surf. In a few seconds the little one will be dipping his toes into the salty water.

His mother, grandfather and I, his Gramma Jo, are witness to the little boy who is about to experience an extraordinary change in his young life. We're seeing for the first time an ocean that has always been there. We stand on the edge of time, as an event that will become etched into our memories unfolds before us.

Our children and grandson are visiting us at our southern vacation home. We have had the amazing experience of sharing many firsts with our grandson over the past few days. Seeing the magic of first times through his innocent eyes has been an honour and a pleasure.

It's a wondrous moment when we adults suddenly see something as if for the first time, even though we have seen it many times before. The difference is, it's through the magic of a little six year old's innocent first experience.

As an ostomate I am still amazed that I have a second chance at life. I am in awe of the power of life itself. Thanks to the creation of my stoma, "Percy", I have the good fortune to live on and experience more of life. Having an ostomy is a daily challenge indeed, and yet, is a great life learning experience. One of the many lessons it teaches me is; life is what we make of it. One can go through it and let things pass them by, or a person can actually go out and capture life as though each moment is the magical first time. And, as life will have it from time to time, when things are especially tough, then we can choose to simply roll with the tide.

Jo-Ann L. Tremblay
Ostomate
"Everyone you meet has a story to tell."

Earth to Jo-Ann…Come In Jo-Ann –
March 19, 2015

It's March 12th and we're so excited. It's 10:34 p.m., we're situated along Florida's Space Coast, (east side of the state on the Atlantic Ocean, 74 kilometres [46 miles], south of Cape Canaveral). The United Launch Alliance Atlas V rocket is at the Space Launch Complex 41 at Cape Canaveral Air Force Station, and is ready for take-off. It's the 4th rocket launch since we arrived here on January 1st.

During the 10 minute countdown to lift off, my imagination kicks in and it brings me back to our home up north, to our bedroom, and to the large photograph hanging over the headboard. It is the now famous photo of planet Earth taken on December 7, 1972, by the crew of the Apollo 17 space-craft, at a distance of about 45,000 kilometres (28,000 mi) from earth, titled, *The Blue Marble*, that I purchased sometime in the 1980's at Kennedy Space Centre.

I bought this photo then because I love our home planet. I find myself often, sitting on my bed and losing myself in the magnificent beauty of our planet. I contemplate our blue jewel suspended in the velvety blackness. I marvel at our fragile sphere.

I think back to 1992 when Roberta Bondar, Canada's first female astronaut boarded the space shuttle *Discovery*, and broke the mould. I recall an interview upon her return from space, she remarked that she had looked out of the window of the shuttle and was struck by all the empty space around our planet. That we're alone in our part of the universe, she pointed out that it's the only home we have right now, and we need to take care of it.

Earth looks peaceful and harmonious from space, but of course all is not as it appears. Conflicts threaten our very survival. Weapons are poised, ready to annihilate life as we know it at a moments notice; environmental crisis is lurking, and conflicts that are rooted in antiquity abound. Human destiny is unclear, the veneer of civilization is yet exceedingly thin, and our current actions bring sustainability into question.

Oh my, the glow of what looks like the dawn of a new day, fully illuminates the horizon to the north of us. It's 10:44 p.m., and we have lift off. Within seconds a large fire ball climbs through the inky black sky. WOW! The rocket has a quartet payload of what is called Magnetospheric Multi-Scale (MMS) spacecraft, which is the first space mission dedicated to the study of magnetic reconnection. My own very basic understanding of magnetic reconnection is that it is a fundamental process that occurs throughout the universe where magnetic fields connect and disconnect with an explosive release of energy. Magnetic reconnection is one of the most important drivers of space weather events, such as eruptive solar flares.

It's amazing to think the journey it took human-kind to arrive at a day where representatives of earth can leave our home planet, not knowing what they will find.

Arriving back to our Florida condo after witnessing the spectacular liftoff I am in awe as I think of humanity's epic journey out of Africa, the cradle of humanity, to eventually populate the earth. We are a species of brave pioneers and adaptive innovators.

I've lived most of my life so far in the 20th century. Those of us who have lived during this time in our planetary history have witnessed the extraordinary miracles and folly of humankind first hand. Ours has been a century of demystifying, human-made miracles and human-made catastrophe. My mother who is only 22 years older than I, lives with the effects of a world evolved from the dim years of the Great Depression to World War 11, and she witnessed the incandescent Nuclear Age.

Progress has been swift for the most part and severe. I have lived through the silent war that was never overtly fought, (Cold War). Watched as humans fought over ideology, and are engaged in an era of organized global terrorism, the likes of which has never before been experienced.

In this age of miracles such as; The Human Genome Project and gene therapy, Pandemic Planning and Coordination of Response, creation of life saving and life sustaining ostomies. The Human Brain Project, an international team of researchers led by German and Canadian scientists have produced a three-dimensional atlas of the brain that has 50 times the resolution of previous maps. Microscale 3-D Printing. And, the list goes on. In my lifetime I have seen the horse drawn ice wagon, delivering ice to my neighbours in a time when not all folks had a refrigerator. And then, just a few years ago my life was saved and extended by the technology of modern medicine, and the skills of medical practitioners.

I have lived momentous days, extraordinary in the ability of people to coordinate their minds and skills to ensure the continuation of humanity's journey and our own individual journeys. The little blue speck in the midst of the vast emptiness that is dotted by luminous celestial bodies is our home, and this ostomate is honoured to be graced with an extended life and the opportunity to live life to the fullest on this beautiful blue marble.

Jo-Ann L. Tremblay
Ostomate
"Everyone you meet has a story to tell."

Breathe – *April 22, 2015*

One day, one moment, one breath at a time. Oh my, I'm pulling air painfully down my throat, to the place where my body is going into spasms of violent coughs. Throat constricted, airways inflamed, each breath a struggle. March was a tough month as I battled an upper respiratory infection. With each effort to breathe, I was reminded of the powerful gift of breath that I had come to realize in the year before Percy Stoma was created. Following is an excerpt from **"Better With A Bag Than In A Bag"**, *From the brink of death to recovery through humour and inspiration*, the book I authored that chronicles my illness that led to colon surgery, Percy's creation, and the year of recovery that followed.

In 2008, when my illness and pain had become chronic, there were times when I was only able to take life one day at a time. Through the years that followed, I was eventually reduced to coping with my body and life one moment at a time. During these times, I often found myself searching, trying to find any reason, any excuse, to have a positive attitude, a positive outlook. I, of course, could find many. I am very fortunate to be blessed in so many ways. But as time advanced along with the illness, I realized that I was not being totally honest with myself in thinking I was being positive while knowing in my heart that I was downright miserable. My mind was in a push-me-pull-me mode. I endured the physical pain as I was drowning in an emotional quagmire. I was sick, angry, and fighting for my quality of life.

As the illness progressed, I arrived at the realization that I was taking life one breath at a time now. It was becoming more and more challenging to remain honestly positive so I decided there must be another way. I could try to talk myself into "positive thinking" until I was blue in the face, but in reality there came the understanding that this approach, this life tool, was not working for me anymore. It was not the appropriate tool for this circumstance. It was not real. It was a mask. It was dishonest. It was downright denial. I needed to step down into the depths of my current reality with eyes wide open. Be truthful with myself. I had to look the monster of my illness and predicament in the eye, with full awareness.

Aha! Awareness. That's the ticket! I began to insert awareness as a coping tool, rather than positive thinking more often than not. In my attempts to simply be aware in the very breaths I took, I used this tool to help develop a deeper understanding of my individuality and the many aspects of myself, my illness, and the life all around me. With full awareness focused and interwoven into each breath, I eventually became sensitive to the truths I was operating from, those I was expressing, and the true realities of my situation. It was honesty, not a fantasy in all its wonder and all of its ugliness. A value-added bonus to this approach was an immersion into the fullness of breath. With every inhale and exhale I realized that time expanded on occasion to the place of forever. I was beyond positive thinking and had arrived at a place where I realized that any one of us can die at any time. It could be today, it could be tomorrow, or in twenty years from now – who really knows? The only thing that is true is that the "now", the "present", is the reality that exist. It is up to us to put as much into and receive as much as possible from that breath, that moment, that day. I was hurting in all ways possible, so it was hard to see a positive future, but it was easy to immerse into my breath and explore the depths, wonders, and potentials a breath can hold. Like a string of pearls, my string of breaths encircled me with the hope and the strength that life – at least for the moment – continued.

I live in awareness because I could die today, tomorrow, or in twenty years from now. I really don't know. Awareness as a tool works for all times, circumstances and situations during the course of a lifetime. Positive thinking is a great tool, one that is appropriate when we are working hard and anticipating a successful outcome. Positive thinking is a tool of great usefulness, but it is not the only tool in our personal and professional toolbox.

Sitting on my patio on those warm summer days during my recovery, I found myself looking back, and looking forward. Awareness is a valuable tool I use quite regularly and continue to hone as my life continues to unfold.

Breath.....breath.....just breath.

Jo-Ann L. Tremblay
Ostomate
"Everyone you meet has a story to tell."

Jo-Ann & Her Bear Hugs – *May 26, 2015*

All good stories begin with *once upon a time*, and so, once upon a time, *there was a lady, her name is Jo-Ann.*

It came to be that I entered into Jo-Ann's life in 2011, during a life saving surgery. You see, I'm part of Jo-Ann's colostomy and since then, I have rocked her world. I'm affectionately known as Percy Stoma, and I fancy myself as her constant companion, I go everywhere she goes.

Stomas will brrt,
and pfft,
and flurppppp,
and thwerrpppp.

(Stomas can make dramatic noises just so everyone knows something is happening down there.)

In the beginning when I first joined her life adventure, our journey was stormy. She did not understand why I had entered her life, nor what I was all about. I was as new to being her stoma, as she was having a colostomy. It took both of us quite awhile to settle in and accept one another. From the very start, as we anticipated our new life together, we were delighted, filled with promise, and hope. At the same time we were frightened, unsure, and lost.

There were many moments, hours and days, we felt we were standing on a pillar of blood red stone, as gun metal black, indigo and grey clouds, swirled and boiled within us. Bolts of lightening cracked and electrified Jo-Ann's mind, as thunder rumbled and exploded throughout our body. The pain and the ecstasy of being alive transcended our spirit. There was no doubt, powerful forces were at work within, as we continued our journey.

Time went by, and we got on with Jo-Ann's life. She made friends who also have stomas. Jo-Ann and I have become familiar with one another, and together we've enjoyed many adventures. We have attended weddings, we've welcomed grand babies, and, as we strive to embrace life, we are slowly and surely learning how to appreciate each other.

It is not always easy. Sometimes we move to the dance of our lives together, and sometimes we are opposed to each other. We are constantly designing our partnership for life. Over time, Jo-Ann has regained her confidence as she encircles me with my ostomy flange. She lovingly surrounds me with a protective pouch. I feel like it's all a great big bear hug!

I, Percy Stoma will brrt,
and pfft,
and flurppppp,
and thwerrpppp.

(Just so everyone knows something is happening down there.)

And, as every good story ends with, and they lived happily every after, when you get a determined ostomate with a fire in her belly and a clever Percy Stoma, they get together and they live happily ever after.

The End

Percy Stoma, Eol. Poopology (**Experience Of** Life)
"Better With A Bag Than In A Bag"

Marching To The Beat Of The Recovery Drum – *June 25, 2015*

June has been a gripping bad news, good news month. A month that held me firmly at attention. It all started with a battle with congestion, which then progressed to become an upper respiratory infection. I am now taking antibiotics and if they work, by next week July 1st, Percy and I will be feeling much better. Not that I should be counting the days, but alas, I am counting the days to a full recovery.

That was the bad news, now for the good news. When one is ill with what may be a contagious germ and everyone stays away from you, what does a writer do with their time, well, they write. Percy and I are so pleased to announce we have completed the manuscript for the sequel to **Better With A Bag Than In A Bag – From the brink of death to recovery through humour and inspiration**, it is now in the hands of our Editor. Percy and I are so excited! Percy has co-written the sequel with me, my clever little stoma. With Percy's sense of humour, straight from the hip no-nonsense, (or in Percy's case, straight from the abdomen, south, south-east, of my belly button), tell it like it is attitude, well, we've had an amazing writing adventure.

Better With A Bag Than In A Bag is a book that shines the light on the odyssey that I was forced to embark on in 2008, that continued to my lifesaving surgery July 21, 2011, and then beyond through the year long recovery afterwards. This book is the real-life story of an ordinary woman taking a stand against an extraordinary nemesis called diverticular disease. The story follows me as I navigated through a myriad of doctors, diagnostic tests, and procedures, only to find myself lost in the mysterious landscape of misdiagnosis. During this time I wondered who would help me. I asked myself many times; "How was I going to save my life before time would run out?"

My life was saved, Percy Stoma was created, and my little buddy has now joined me on this journey called life. The first book chronicles my march to the beat of the recovery drum, and the many bizarre, often times comic, definitely frustrating, and challenging situations and circumstances an ostomate faces. It is a book that I shared the poop on poops as a new ostomate, with humour, and the triumph of the human spirit that is within all of us. I have had the pleasure of receiving emails and letters from readers, many of which are ostomates, and others who are not. One of the most often shared comment I receive is, *"This book made me laugh, and made me cry, it provided me with vital information, and it gave me hope."* Another ostomate comment is, *"This book made me remember my own journey from the brink, and it has inspired me to continue taking those small steps forward."* Percy and I are so very pleased that in sharing our story, we have been valuable for so many.

On the day of my first stomaversary, we enjoyed friends, good eats, and all of the sparkle July 21, 2012, could bring. On July 22, 2012, the following day, the full impact of reality set in and I realized that although the official recovery period was now completed, Percy and I found ourselves at a "beginning again". Hmm…Well, ah, the beginning of what, who, when, where and how, of a new life, new self, and a new normal, whatever the heck it's all supposed to be. And so, the *sequel* begins the day after our first Celebration of Life Stomaversary Day, where Better With A Bag Than In A Bag, ends. The candles had been blown out, the cupcakes devoured. Percy and I had thrown away our gem-studded ostomy pouch. Time to move on – or so we thought.

Living with the full impact of the lingering damage from the original disease and the damage from the extensive surgery. Coupled, with the emotional toll it takes to adapt and live with an altered body function, and another surgery about to be scheduled, on the horizon there was another storm brewing. Gun metal black, indigo, and grey clouds of pain and doubt swirled and boiled, inside of me. My body and emotions seemed filled with unseen monsters, bewitching me with their seductive mystery, beckoning ever beckoning me to jump. With all that was in Percy and I, it was time for us to harness the power of the storm within.

The *sequel*, chronicles the 2nd year march to the beat of our recovery drum. Together, with an army of family, friends, caregivers and medical professionals, we navigated through our healing journey that has been filled with disaster and triumph. This is my individualized true life tale of exploration and adventure as I perceive it. An adventure that goes beyond survival to arrive at the gateway of a new world, a new life, a new normal.

Through THE OSTOMY FACTOR blog, Twitter, and Facebook, Percy and I are pleased to keep you up to date on the latest announcements, notifications, and the publication date of: **Another Bag, Another Day – *creating a new lease on life in a new world***.

Jo-Ann L. Tremblay   &   Percy Stoma
Ostomate   Eol. in Poopology
  "Everyone you meet has a story to tell."

Stomaversary! - *July 21, 2015*

Happy stomaversary to us, happy stomaversary to us, happy stomaversary dear Percy and Jo-Ann. Happy stomaversary to us.

Wow Jo-Ann, it's our stomaversary. Sounds like party time to me.

Yes Percy, it's our 4th year together. It sure has been an experience and a half little buddy.

A lot of water has passed under the bridge as they say, during this time. Percy Stoma and I embarked on our adventure together on July 21, 2011. It was a crazy time for us. I had arrived at hospital in such a condition that the attending physician stated that if I was to have arrived an hour later, the odds on me surviving were slim to none. During the lifesaving surgery, Percy was created and I must say my life hasn't been the same since.

"Hey, I hope that's a compliment", Jo-Ann.

"It sure is, I would not be alive without you Percy, you're my hero."

"Oh I like that, I'm a hero!"

"Of course living with a stoma is not always easy, you are high maintenance, little buddy."

"I guess living with a hero has its price, Jo-Ann."

"Yes, I suppose it does"

At any rate, a lot of living sure has happened throughout the past 4 years. During the first year of recovery Percy and I had to adjust to one another. Relationships of every kind takes a lot of hard work, and stomas are not an exception. Then, during the following year we underwent another major surgery. As time passed during those years, the good news is; Percy has taken care of the elimination end of things, and I've regained control of my life.

After our ostomies are created, an ostomate must then continue to live with the ravages left behind from the original disease, and there is always the complications from these invasive surgeries. To add to the experience, there are the ongoing everyday physical and psychological realities of living with an altered bio elimination system and required equipment. Let's just say there are many bumps on the road. An ostomates life, is a life that is forever changed. Many of us feel we are living another life, in another world. The fact of the matter is; we are living another life and it sure is another world for us. It is our second opportunity, it's another chance to live, to laugh, to cry, to struggle, to triumph, and another chance to live life to the fullest.

There is a time in everyone's life when something important to us is lost. Then, there is the time when we really and truly notice the loss. We enter into upset, denial, we can even feel anger, and we grieve our loss. We experience the difficult moments when we remember what we lost, and we want to go back to the time before our loss for a visit. We strive to make peace with what has happened. Then, we explore what we can do about it all, so that we can come out to the other side.

Starting July 22, 2011, Percy and I chose to keep on moving through our lives in spite of ourselves, and it was me who was to get us both moving somewhere. We know we're not broken for good, nor are we beyond repair, of sorts. It's terrible what's happened to us, and there are so many brave people and stomas out there going through their own struggles and tragedies. For sure I'm sorry that all of this happened to me, but I'm an active spirit, and both Percy and I decided after a couple of years together, that we'd take on the attitude that we could turn this around and use our challenges for the sake of ourselves and others. We decided that from tragedy that we'd create elation. I've often heard it said; "tragedy and elation are often close neighbours", and so, our work began.

I promised Percy we would start again as we go along on this life journey, and together we made commitments. We've committed to ostomy awareness, to be advocates where needed, and we will share all that we experience and learn with all, in various ways and forms within our abilities, skills, and energy. We have set out to learn everything we can about ostomies, ostomates, how to cope, accept, manage, and learn how to live as an ostomate in partnership with our little stoma buddies. This journey has taken us beyond basic survival to a place where we feel we are flourishing.

With our commitment in mind, in 2012 Percy and I created, **THE OSTOMY FACTOR** blog. In that same year I wrote and published, **Better With A Bag Than In A Bag**, for more information, go to the menu bar at the top of this page and click Better With A Bag Than In A Bag. Percy and I have co-authored the sequel, **Another Bag, Another Day**, which will be published and available for purchase from Amazon, the the fall of 2015.

In 2013, Better With A Bag Than In A Bag, was reviewed and the review article was featured in *The Phoenix Magazine*, The official publication of the United Ostomy Association of America.

In the winter of 2014, Percy and I were featured on the cover of *Tidings Magazine*, and "Jo-Ann's second chance at life....", was the inside Cover story. Tidings Magazine is released every quarter, each issue of Tidings contains real life stories, features on Ostomate issues, updates from the Colostomy Association – UK, the latest products and more. www.colostomyassociation.org.uk.

Also in 2014, as part of our quest to support ostomy awareness and advocacy, I became a member of the *Medical Advisory Committee* with the *Ostomy Canada Society*. The Ostomy Canada Society is a non-profit volunteer organization dedicated to all people with an ostomy, and their families/friends, helping them to live life to the fullest through support, education, collaboration and advocacy.

As a member of the Medical Advisory Committee, my area of responsibility is *Ostomy Lifestyle Expert*, (www.ostomycanada.ca) In this capacity, I respond to questions posed by the general public on a variety of ostomy relate subjects. Go to the very well designed and information filled Ostomy Canada Society website. To enjoy the Ostomy Lifestyle Expert page, click on "Information" on the websites bar at the top of the page, a pop menu will appear, click on *"Ask an Ostomy Lifestyle Expert"*. Together we are learning so much.

In addition, Percy and I have enjoyed writing articles published in the *OstomyCanada Magazine*. This quality, full colour magazine is published twice a year, and offers ostomy related information as well as motivational personal stories, and up-to-date product information, it is a valuable publication to be enjoyed by all.

Over the past several years Percy and I have had the pleasure of being invited as *Guest Speaker* in the United States and Canada. It sure has been a delight to meet and share in fellowship, with the *Ostomy Support Groups*, we've made many ostomate and stoma friends.

On a personal note, during the past 4 years Percy and I have witnessed the birth of 3 of our 6 grandchildren. We have filled our lives with all of them, as they grow and develop into their own. We had the pleasure of enjoying a daughter's wedding, and are now anticipating the birth of her first child, our 7th grandchild. We have travelled on many adventures, and have met many new friends.

"Well Percy, we've been busy living, laughing, crying, struggling, we've had our triumphs and our failures, but through it all, we're living our life to the fullest."

"Yes, we sure have been busy, just as we like it. I'd like to add something here Jo-Ann?"

"Sure Percy."

"Ahem...Thank you to everyone who has come on this journey with us, and may your next year ahead be the best yet."

Jo-Ann L. Tremblay, Ostomate
Percy Stoma, Eol. Poopology
"Everyone we meet has a story to tell."

The Art of Life & The Life of Art – *August 11, 2015*

It is the supreme art of the teacher to awaken joy in creative expression and knowledge – Albert Einstein.

It was my distinct honour and pleasure to enjoy an art day with our 10 year old granddaughter Emelyn, in July. Oh, what a glorious day! We immersed ourselves in the logistics of preparing for our art, acquiring the necessary tools to create with, and the joy of creating. Emelyn explored and engaged in every aspect of the creative process. She had so many wonderful questions. For example; "What medium is best for what I want to accomplish?"

Together we explored the art store shelves filled with paint brushes, as I shared information on the various painting tools an artist would use in order to achieve a particular technique and outcome. Then we chose the type and size canvas shapes to compliment the paint medium to be used, and for the display configuration she envisioned for her art creations on the wall. We took a time out, enjoying our lunch together, as we explored and discussed her art project ideas.

Arriving home we immersed into creating. We laughed and giggled with the joy of our imaginations as she worked all afternoon breathing life into 3 canvases. She transformed each plain white canvas into colourful vistas of beauty that evoke the emotional power of creativity and imagination. When we completed the final canvas she exclaimed, "I love this one, look how the colours blended!"

Her art shimmers with colourful creative expression, and at the same time the art anchors the accomplishment of, "I created this." Her loving and supportive family have honoured her artistic pieces by displaying them. One is on the dinning-room wall, one in the living-room, and the third at the front door. Everyone who enters their home is graced with the opportunity to appreciate each work and to explore them with their own individual imagination.

The life of art is the application and expression of our human creative energy and imagination. It is an exploration enjoyed by the artist and the viewer alike. Stirring the imagination, the art invites them to explore their own revelations from within the art, each time it is viewed.

The art of life engages us in envisioning what is important to us, and what we want for and from our life experience. Initially without knowing all of the details of what, when, where and the how of what we are choosing, we immerse ourselves into the logistics of preparing for our artful life vision. We inventory our tools in the form of talents, skills and abilities, in our personal and professional toolbox that we will use to make our vision become reality. If we don't have a particular tool to achieve a particular outcome, then we explore what is required and we acquire that tool, all for the purpose of creating. We choose what we want our vision to look like, and then, where and how it will fit into the canvas of our lives.

Time outs on our own and with others are important interludes for rest and relaxation, which is always helpful in bringing forward the appreciation of our current reality, as we explore the hopes and dreams of our visualized future.

We immerse ourselves in living and working on ourselves and on our life experiences. We laugh and we cry as we breathe life into the blank canvas of our lives. We transform ourselves and our lives with the emotional power of our creativity and imagination. Even those whose point of view is that they and/ or their lives are mundane, can say, "This didn't just happen, I created this, at least in some part." Even if they are not creating everything that is showing up or not showing up, as the case may be in their life, somehow they are contributing something to it.

In art and in life, you are always using your point of view paint brush. Some of us choose to transform ourselves and lives into technicolor creations. Some of us choose to transform the technicolor of our lives into black and white creations.

In life and in art, with every blank canvas, regardless of any and all happenings, there is always the hope that our creative expressions and the knowledge we gain through our choices, that there will always be constant generation and creation of possibilities.

In the life of art and in the art of life, the artist takes control of their visions, the self, and their tools as they immerse into every creative and life expression. What the artist cannot control, they then use the experience as an inspiration. Neither the artist nor the art is perfect, this leaves room for them to further develop and grow. In the experiences of the artist, life is an ongoing process of discovery and co-creation with life.

Jo-Ann L. Tremblay
Ostomate
"Everyone you meet has a story to tell."

Jo-Ann's New Book – Another BAG Another DAY – *September 23, 2015*

Jo-Ann's Latest Book, **Another Bag, Another Day**, is the sequel to **Better With A Bag Than In A Bag**. Jo-Ann an ostomate and Percy her life sustaining stoma have co-written this funny, hopeful, yet inspirational and adventurous true life account of their journey as they march to the beat of the recovery drum. With all the power left in them, this story goes beyond survival to arrive at the gateway of a new world, a new life, a new normal.

Jo-Ann's New Book

Another Bag, Another Day

Arrives September 23, 2015

After September 23rd you can order your Kindle & Paper Back copies through Amazon (Canada, USA, UK, Europe, Australia, Mexico, France, Germany, Italy, Spain, India, China)

EXTRA...EXTRA...Another BAG Another DAY has arrived! *September 15, 2015*

Percy and I are pleased to announce: **Another BAG Another Day** *Creating a new Lease on Life in a New World* (the sequel to *Better WITH a Bag Than IN a Bag*), is now available **in paperback and KINDLE versions**. Soon to come on KOBO and iTUNES

NOW AVAILABLE ON AMAZON

CELEBRATING WORLD OSTOMY DAY –
October 3, 2015

An estimated 750,000 Americans and 90,000 Canadians live with an ostomy every day, including myself. Our ostomies have saved our lives and now we have a 2nd chance at living life to the fullest. Through awareness and advocacy we are celebrating all who have and will have an ostomy, and to the families, friends, caregivers, and medical professionals, who will join them on their journey.

Live, love, laugh and enjoy your day to the fullest!

Percy and I send our best to you all.

7 Bursts of Glow – *October 7, 2015*

Oh how wondrous, it's pure delight! Seven is a number that is often referred to as the number of completeness and perfection, (both physical and spiritual). There are 7 days of the week, 7 notes of the musical scale, and 7 directions (left, right, up, down, forward, back and centre). And for us, 7 also represents the birth of our 7th grandchild. So tiny and so innocent, our little granddaughter has the magical ability to ignite us with a burst of glow that glimmers and gleams. She is snuggled up within us and the radiance of her glow has added to the luminosity of our heart light that now outshines the celestial sun.

A friend of mine recently said, "If we had to do it all over again, we'd probably have our grandchildren first." For me, I am in awe that my life was spared, Percy Stoma was created, and I was carved into a survivor. As an ostomate, this 2nd chance at life means I can live my life to the fullest. As ostomates we have another opportunity to embrace the joy and trials of experiencing our lives as it unfolds.

Already our 7th little one and I have mounted her unicorn (named Stinky), and began our mystical journey through the mushroom fields and peony forests. Arriving at the enchanted grove where the faeries live, one by one each of the faeries sprinkled shimmering faerie glitter on her button nose.

As life will have it, this is the beginning of many adventures we will embark upon together. Her birth is the start of her circle of life, ostomates such as myself have been reborn, and have begun another circle of life.

Welcome little one to the Planet and to your time. May you live life to the fullest.

Welcome *ALL* who create a 2nd chance at life, may you once and again live life to the fullest.

Jo-Ann L. Tremblay
Ostomate
"Everyone you meet has a story to tell"

Every Tomorrow Has Two Handles – *November 24, 2015*

Every tomorrow has two handles. We can take hold of it with one handle of anxiety or the handle of faith. – Henry Ward Beecher

Living with a chronic physical, emotional and/or mental health issue is like perpetually riding a roller coaster for the first time. When we have a flare up of any sort we feel the rapid reversal of direction and that can be scary because of the unknown ahead in our highly dynamic individual health environment.

When the reversal hits, its like the feeling you get in an auto accident. Everything appears in ultra-slow motion as you see the oncoming vehicle. You're powerless to move. All you can do is get that sick feeling in your stomach when you know the pain is about to strike, and there is nothing you can do about it. Then, the excruciating painful reality hits you hard...full force...WHAM!

On the roller coaster, once we realize the ups are always followed by the downs and visa versa, and we can see the snaking of the track ahead of us, then we can begin to anticipate the next inevitable reversal and brace ourselves for it.We know we won't be able to avoid it, but with each reversal we become more accustomed to the sudden changes, pulls, and drops.

When my ostomy, was created, it was during emergency life-saving surgery. When I awakened from the 8 hour surgery I found that I was now an ostomate. I had no idea what an ostomy was. I had no clue about what was required to take care of myself, nor how to care for my ostomy.

At that pivotal point in my life I had been permanently physiologically altered, and so, was inevitably emotionally and mentally altered. I didn't know what to think, how to behave, nor how I was going to go forward in life. I didn't even know what the new me was, let alone how to be the new me.

Everyone has their individualized life issue(s), in my case I am an ostomate. It has taken years of research through;

• connecting with fellow ostomates

• joining a local ostomy support group

• becoming a member of ostomy social media groups

• following ostomy websites, newsletters, blogs

• and, meeting with Enterostomal Therapists (ET Nurses).

Through my research and connections, after 4 years I now for the most part feel the confidence in knowing I am no longer blindfolded as I live my ostomy roller coaster ride.

Through knowledge and better understanding of our chronic life/health issue(s), we are able to rip away the blindfold, as we live with the perpetual knowing that as the days, weeks and months go by the next gut-wrenching reversal of direction will occur. That's the emotional character of the experienced person with chronic life/health issues.

Whatever life/health issue you live, whatever community of humanity you choose, and through whatever medium that works for you, know that; through connecting with like minded people who can relate and live the same issues as you do, (and there are many-you are not alone), you will feel the support. As you give and receive from each other you learn so very much. You will know how to prepare for the worst, and adapt as best you can to the ups and downs.

The key is: adaptation.

We can adapt better when we know what is coming, we learn to know when it might happen, what could possibly bring it on, and we have a plan to adjust to our new normal, our new world.

As every tomorrow unfolds as it will and come what may, we are presented with two handles to choose from, this is the choice for today and for our tomorrow.

Jo-Ann L. Tremblay
Ostomate
"Everyone you meet has a story to tell."

Sand Angels – *December 16, 2015*

Christmas is upon us and the music of the Christmas season is playing on the radio. We sway to the sounds of crackling, crystalline snow. There are songs that transport us to enchanted glacial vistas, sometimes with a jingling tempo, and at other times with songs that bring us to storybook powdery northern vistas. All beautiful as they transport us back in time and space.

We're celebrating our first Christmas south, way south of our pure white Canadian home. As I listen to the music, it really strikes me as to how odd that my head is filled with visions and memories of sparkling snow, while my body is nestled on a sandy beach all warm and glowing in the sparkling sun. What a contrasting effect!

As the radio station is playing **"Sleigh Ride"**, my body is heating up in the sun and my mind is wandering as it often does and I find that I'm changing the words of the song as I sing along to fit my southern experience.

(**Sleigh Ride** *is a piece composed by Leroy Anderson completed in February 1948. Originally an instrumental piece, lyrics, about a person who would like to ride in a sleigh on a winter's day with another person, were written by Mitchell Parish in 1950. The orchestral version was first recorded in 1949 by Arthur Fiedler and the Boston Pops Orchestra. Over the years, the song has become a Christmas standard.)*

So, with a lighthearted celebration of Christmas, here's my version of "Sleigh Ride" that I call, "Sand Angels".

SAND ANGELS

Just hear those beach venders bells jingle-ing
Ring ting tingle-ing too
Come on, it's lovely weather
For making sand angels together with you

Outside the sand is heating up
And friends are calling "Yoo Hoo"
Come on, it's lovely weather
For making sand angels with you

Giddy-yap, giddy-yap, giddy-yap
Let's go
Let's look at the ocean ebb and flow
We're sitting in a wonderland of sand

Giddy-yap, giddy-yap, giddy-yap it's grand
Just holding your hand
We're dancing in our beach chairs with the song
Of a beachy fairyland

Our cheeks are nice and our noses burnt red
And comfy cozy are we
We're snuggled up like two
shore birds of a feather would be

Let's take a walk on the stretch of beach
And sing a chorus or two
Come on, it's lovely weather
For making sand angels together with you

There's a beach party under the sun umbrella at Crusty Crabs
We'll be singing the songs we love to sing without a stop
At the fire pit while we watch popcorn pop
Pop! Pop! Pop!

There's a happy feeling nothing in the world can buy
When they pass around the beer and we swat the flies
It'll nearly be like a picture print of Beach Comber Sy
These wonderful things are the things
We remember all through our lives

We miss our Canadian family and friends, but for this year, we are celebrating the Christmas season with all of its joy and reverence having fun in the sun.

Mark, Percy and I, wish everyone a **MERRY CHRISTMAS** and a **HAPPY NEW YEAR**. May 2016 be the best year yet for **ALL**.

Jo-Ann L. Tremblay – Ostomate
Percy Stoma (Eol. Poopology)
"Everyone you meet has a story to tell."

PS – We are so excited, check our newly re-designed lighthearted and informative website

www.jo-annltremblay.com

About the Author

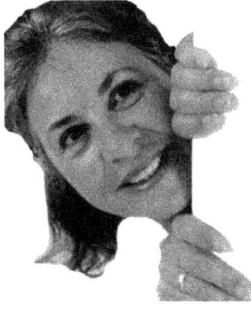

Jo-Ann L. Tremblay is a personal/professional life coach, trainer, photographer, and water colour/oil artist. This is her fourth book. All books are in support of her awareness and advocacy endeavours. Jo-Ann has created and hosted the television special, **That's Life**, hosted two television program series — and a radio program series, **Voices of Our Town**.

After a lengthy illness, Jo-Ann underwent life-saving surgery that resulted in the creation of an ostomy and the stoma she affectionately calls "Percy". Now an ostomate, Jo-Ann L. Tremblay joins with fellow ostomates, their caregivers, medical experts and people in general, through speaking engagements, writing magazine articles, and is a member of the Medical Advisory Committee in the capacity of Ostomy Lifestyle Expert with the Canada Ostomy Society, ostomycanada.ca.

To automatically receive the **THE OSTOMY FACTOR** blog (usually 1 post per month), go to; joannltremblay.wordpress.com. Look to the right hand side panel, there you will see, "Follow Blog via Email". Simply enter your email address to follow the blog and receive notifications of new posts by email.

Website: www.jo-annltremblay.com
Blog: joannltremblay.wordpress.com *(The Ostomy Factor)*
Twitter: @joanntremblay
Facebook: Author Jo-Ann L. Tremblay

Other Books by Jo-Ann L. Tremblay

Better WITH a Bag Than IN a Bag

ISBN-13: 978-0-9809009-1-0

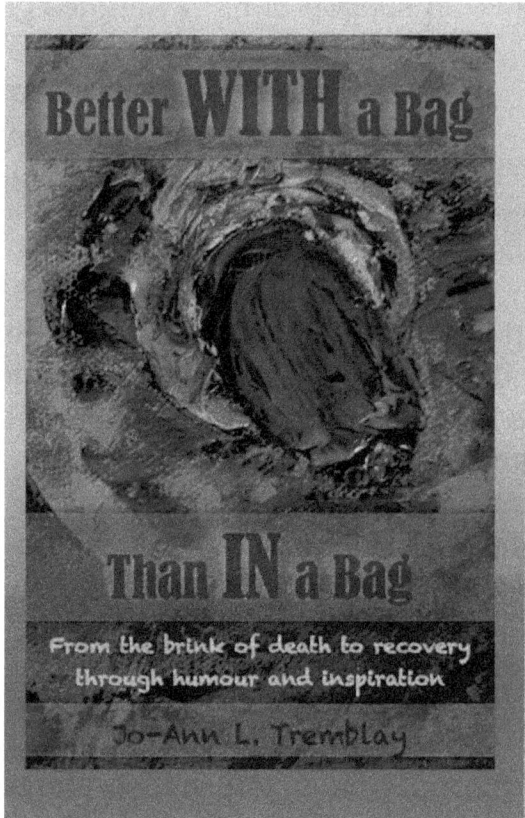

Available on Amazon (PAPERBACK and KINDLE),
throughout the world

As an E-BOOK on iTunes
As an E-BOOK on Kobo

In PAPERBACK at:
Barnes and Noble   Alibris.com or Alibris UK

Another BAG, Another DAY

ISBN-13: 978-0-9809009-2-7

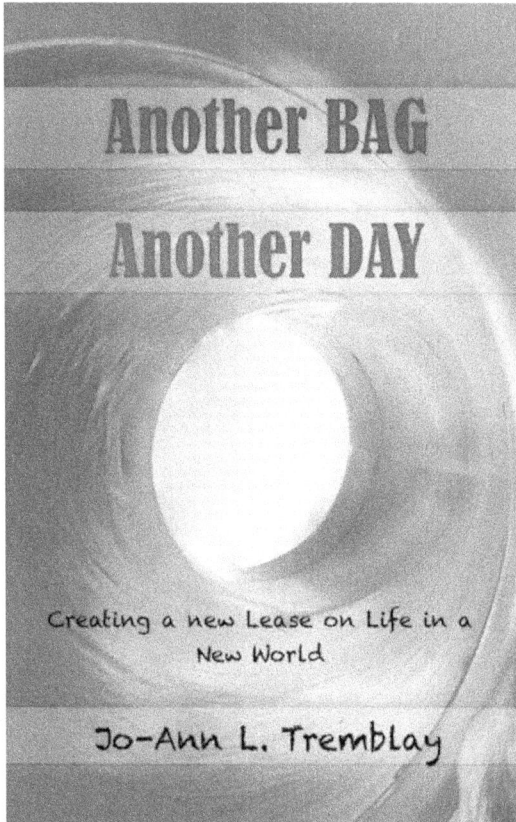

Available on Amazon (PAPERBACK and KINDLE),
throughout the world

As an E-BOOK on iTunes
As an E-BOOK on Kobo

In PAPERBACK at:
Barnes and Noble   Alibris.com or Alibris UK

The Self-Coaching Toolbox
(Original Paperback Edition)

ISBN 1-897113-06-4

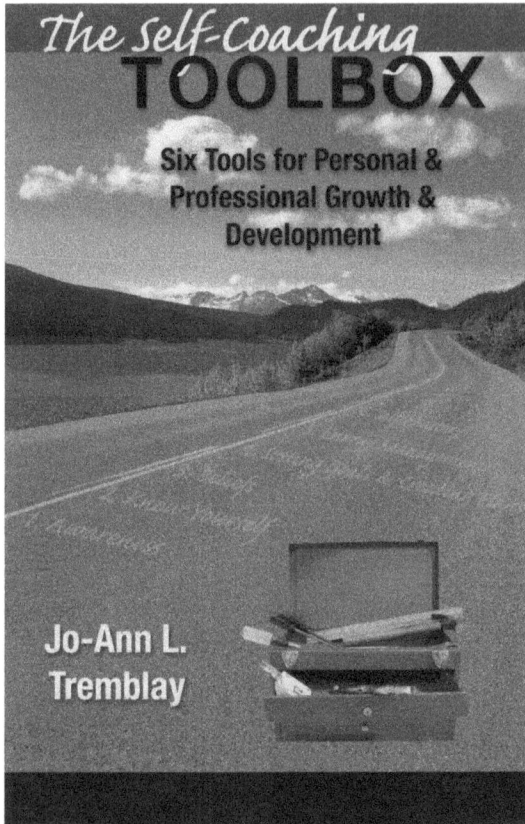

Available
In PAPERBACK at:
Amazon
Alibris.com or Alibris UK

www.ingramcontent.com/pod-product-compliance
Lightning Source LLC
Chambersburg PA
CBHW071125280326
41935CB00010B/1118